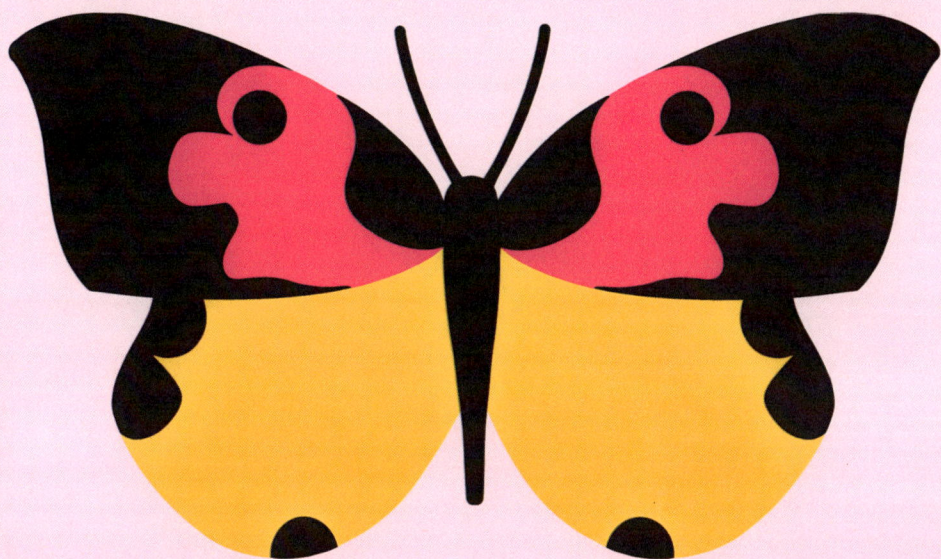

bless my broccoli

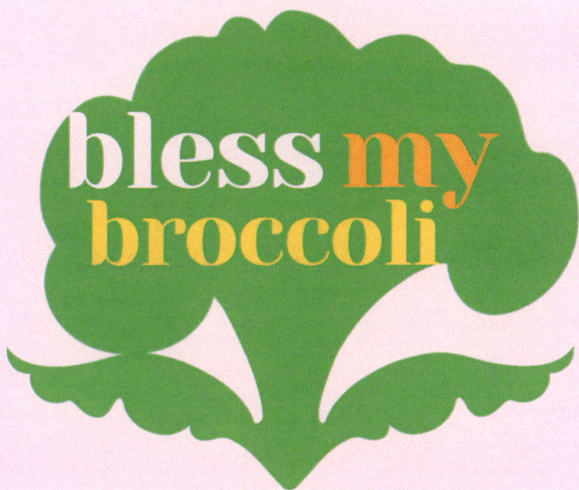

a whole faith, plant-based prayer book for those who want to eat like an angel

Seanra Kalil

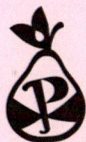

PEARING
PRINTING PRESS
WINNETKA, ILLINOIS

wellnesspatternstudio.com

Wellness Pattern, Inc.
Pearing Printing Press
Winnetka, Illinois, USA

Publisher's Cataloging-in-Publication Data

Names: Kalil, Seanra, author.
Title: Bless my broccoli : a whole faith , plant-based prayer book for those who want to eat like an angel / Seanra Kalil.
Description: Winnetka, IL: Pearing Printing Press, 2025.
Identifiers: LCCN: 2025905250 | ISBN: 979-8-9926635-1-8 (hardcover) | 979-8-9926635-0-1 (ebook)
Subjects: LCSH Vegetables--Poetry. | American poetry--21st century. | Vegan cooking. | Christian poetry. | BISAC POETRY / Subjects & Themes / Religious | RELIGION / Christian Living / General | COOKING / Specific Ingredients / Vegetables | COOKING / Vegan Classification: LCC PS3611 .A55 B54 2025 | DDC 811.6--dc23

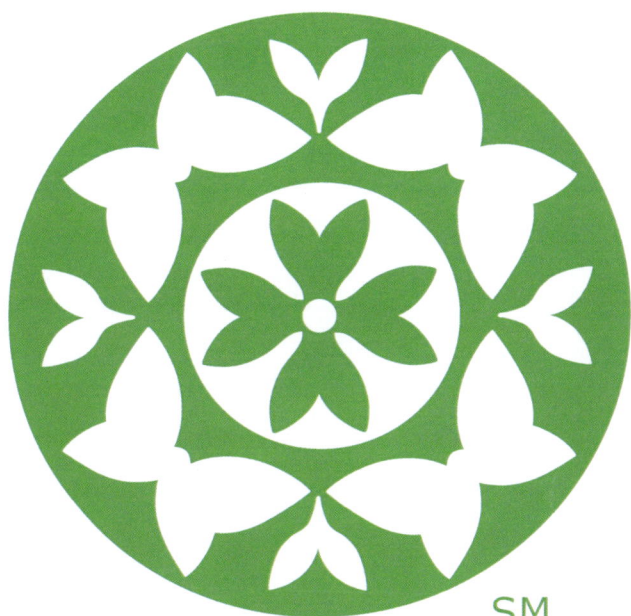

SM

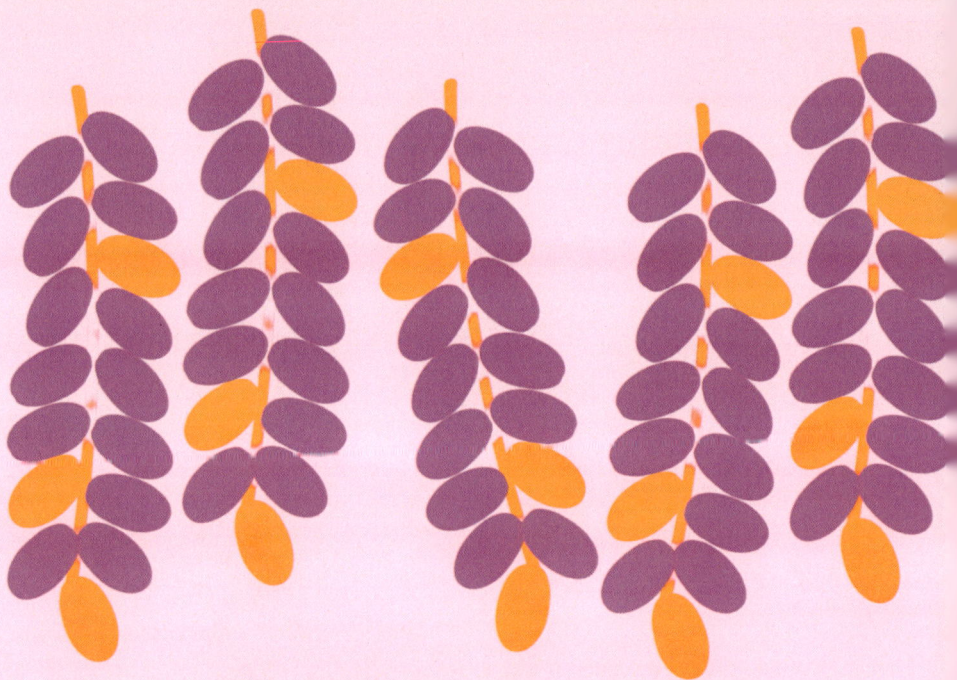

For authors with much expertise:
October dates and mulberries.

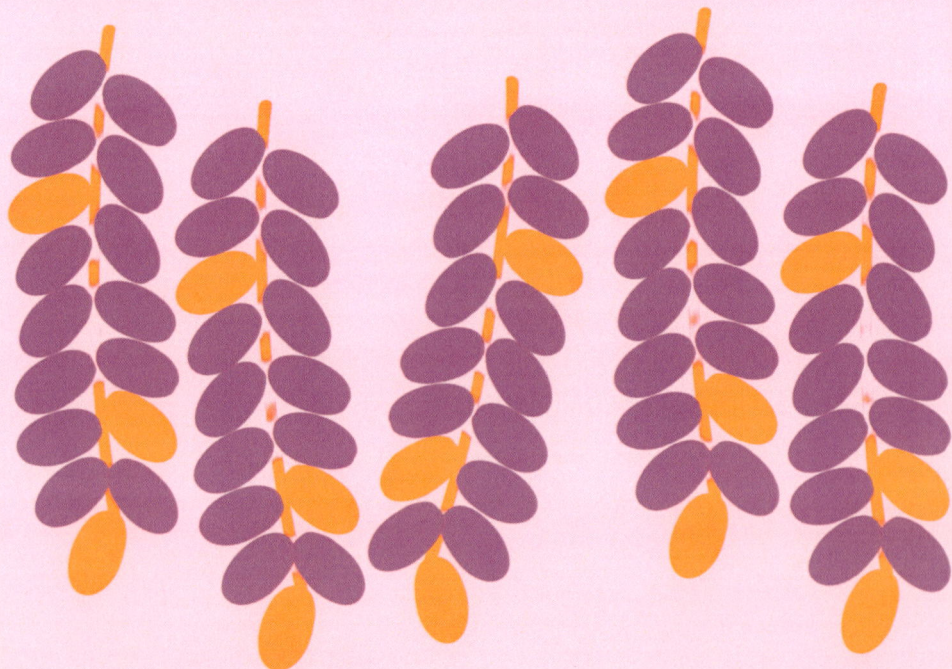

Many many thanks

To Rhonda Byrne,
you are a star that ever sparkles.

To Michael Greger, M.D., FACLM,
you are all healthy foods, and then some.

To our veterans and all who serve in
the United States Armed Forces
—my deepest gratitude.
Your sacrifice makes poetry possible.

yes, it's homemade

Thank you so much for your interest in my book and message: gratitude for real food opens the path to true health and happiness.

The poems you'll see on the following pages began about eight years ago, before AI chatbots came onto the scene. Though I considered "perfecting" my work, I feel it's best left organic, with flaws just like us. Humans are imperfect, and that is what makes us special.

To expand my vocabulary, I read the dictionary. I didn't know that was actually a thing, but it made sense to go to a "word bank." It was a long process, but also quite interesting. Words have so much power. I hope you use your voice in a meaningful and positive way, such as through prayer and blessings.

For the illustrations, I used autofill, the copy-and-paste feature in a basic graphic design program, and relied heavily on the computer's French curves; however, I consider these basic tools. Like reading the dictionary, I did equal research for the art, studying the shapes, colors, and details of each food, often eating them while drawing. Because some are seasonal, I waited many months to complete certain pages.

My intent is to offer you a new perspective on diet, which I truly believe is the most enjoyable way to improve our health. More importantly, it also honors God, who has provided us with everything we could ever need.

drawn by number

In designing these illustrations, I wanted to acknowledge the order God placed in creation. I followed the Fibonacci sequence (0, 1, 1, 2, 3, 5, 8, 13, 21, 34, 55, etc.) when choosing the number of fruits, seeds, vegetables, beans, grains, and/or flowers on each page. The Fibonacci sequence reveals how patterns and growth appear naturally. Did you know that as you move along this sequence, the ratio of each consecutive pair of numbers (such as 34/21 or 55/34) approaches the golden ratio (approximately 1.618)? The more we look, the more we see how wondrous life truly is. I hope this book offers you another way to count your blessings.

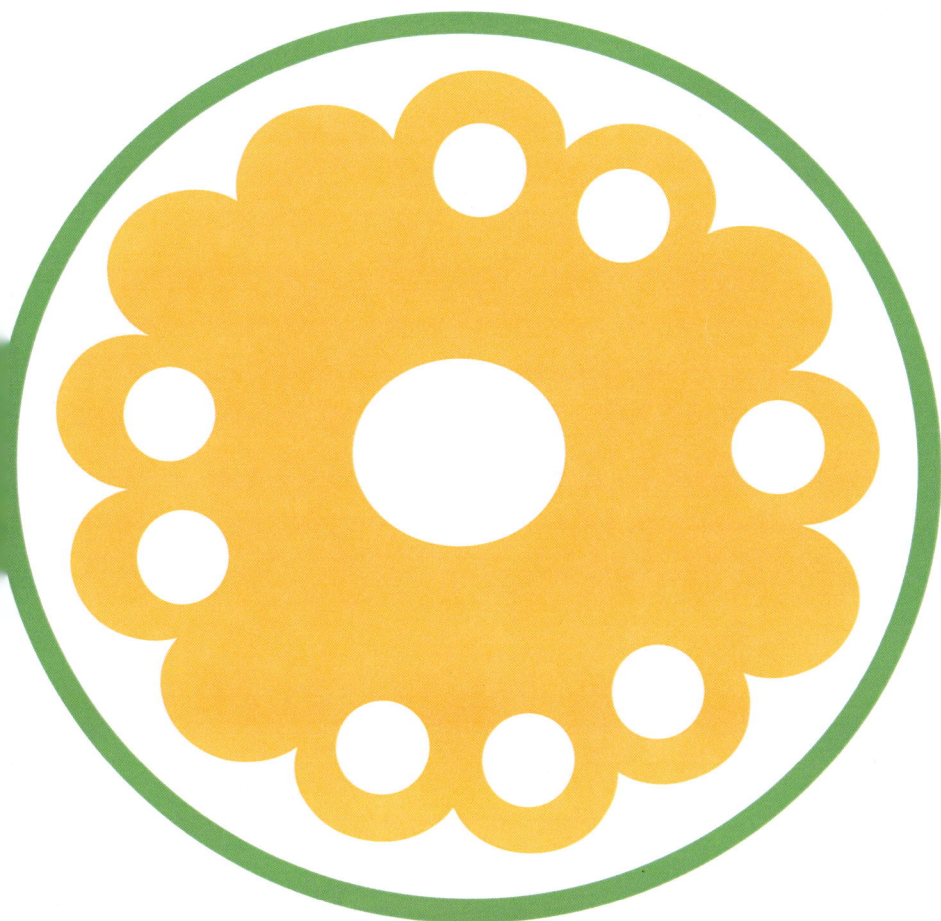

ingredients

Acorn squash
Amla
Apricot
Artichoke
Avocado
Banana
Bartlet pear
Bell pepper
Bing cherry
Black bean
Black plum
Black raspberry
Blood orange
Bok choy
Borage star flower
Bosc pear
Broccoli
Broccoli flower
Butternut squash
Button mushroom
Carrot
Cauliflower
Celery
Celery root
Chamomile
Cherry tomato
Chard
Chia seed
Chive flower
Cilantro
Cranberry bean
Cranberry hibiscus
Cucumber flower
Curly kale
Dates
Dandelion
Day lily
Dill flower
Dragon fruit
Elderberry
Elderflower
Eggplant
Fig and fig leaf
Flax flower
Garbanzo bean
Gem lettuce
Goji berry
Golden apple
Golden beet
Golden oyster mushroom

Gold kiwifruit
Gooseberry
Green grape
Green lentil
Green olive
Ground cherry
Hazelnut
Heirloom tomato
Hollyhock
Honeydew flower bud
Hot pepper
Huckleberry
Jackfruit
Jalapeño pepper
Jasmine
Jicama
Kiwi
Kirby cucumber
Kumquat
Kuri squash
Lemon balm
Lemon guava
Lemon plum
Licorice flower
Lima bean
Lime
Lisbon lemon
Lychee
Mango
Marigold
Meyer lemon
Mulberries
Mustard flower
Mustard seed
Napa cabbage
Nasturtium
Navy bean
Nori seaweed
Oat
Orange
Orange blossom
Orchid
Papaya
Parsley
Passion fruit
Peach
Pecan
Pepino melon
Peppermint
Persimmon
Pineapple
Pink guava

Pinto bean
Pistachio
Pumpkin leaf
Prickly pear
Prune plum
Purple potato
Quince
Quinoa
Rainier cherry
Raspberry
Red delicious apple
Red garden beet
Red grapefruit
Red lentil
Red oak leaf lettuce
Red onion
Red radish
Rose
Rose hip
Rosemary
Roselle hibiscus
Saffron
Sage
Sea lettuce
Snow pea
Soy bean
Spinach
Spring onion
Squash blossom
Star apple
Star fruit
Strawberry
Summer squash
Sunflower
Swamp rose
Sweet corn
Sweet potato
Table grape
Tangerine
Turnip
Vanilla seed pod
Wasabi
Watermelon
White currant
White nectarine
White radish
Wild blueberry
Wood sorrel leaf
Yellow onion
Yellow wax bean
Zinnia
Zucchini

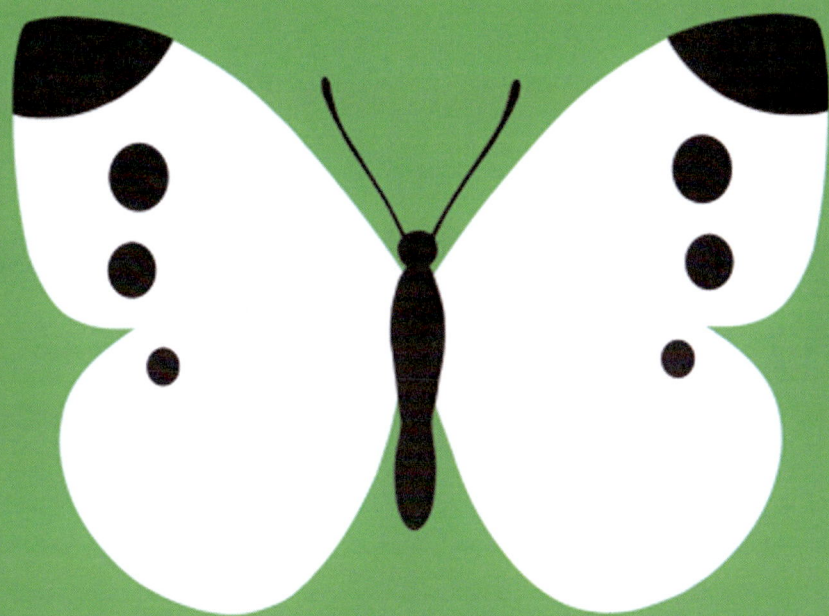

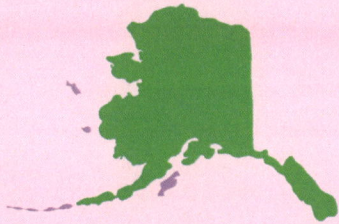

We are praying for our country,
its farm lands, vast fields, and pantries,
from Nevada to New Jersey,
Montana to Mississippi.

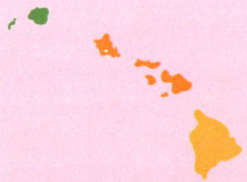

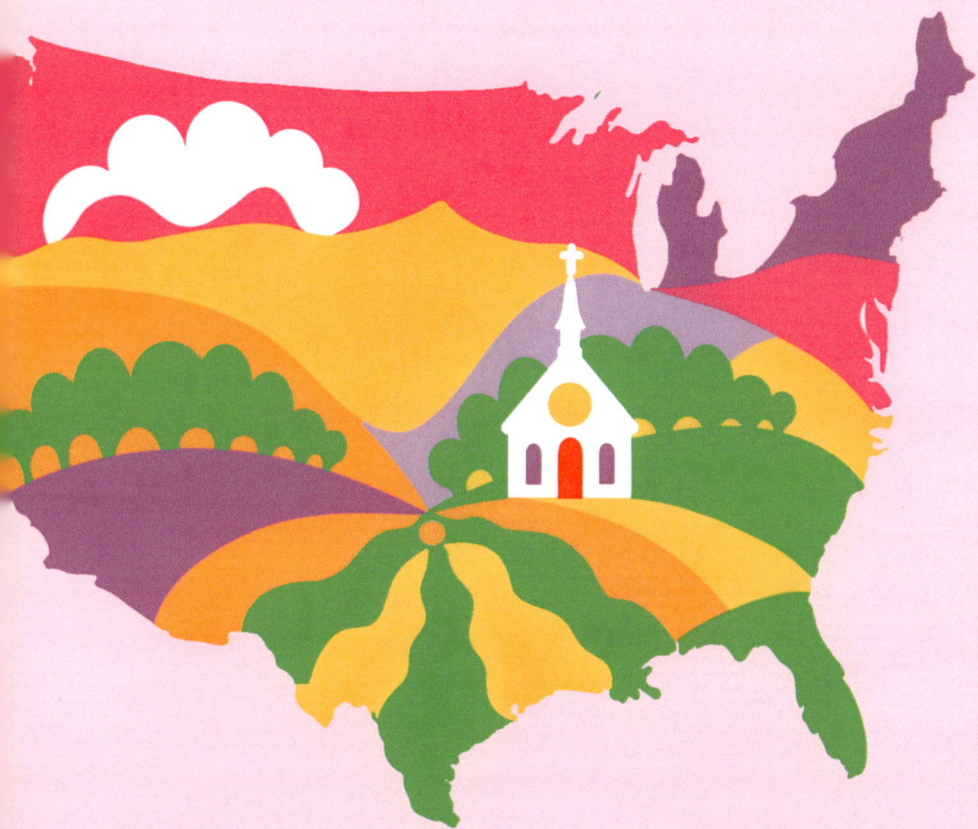

Growing food exceptionally.
All organic, ideally.

Let us focus on what's worthy,
not too late, but always early.

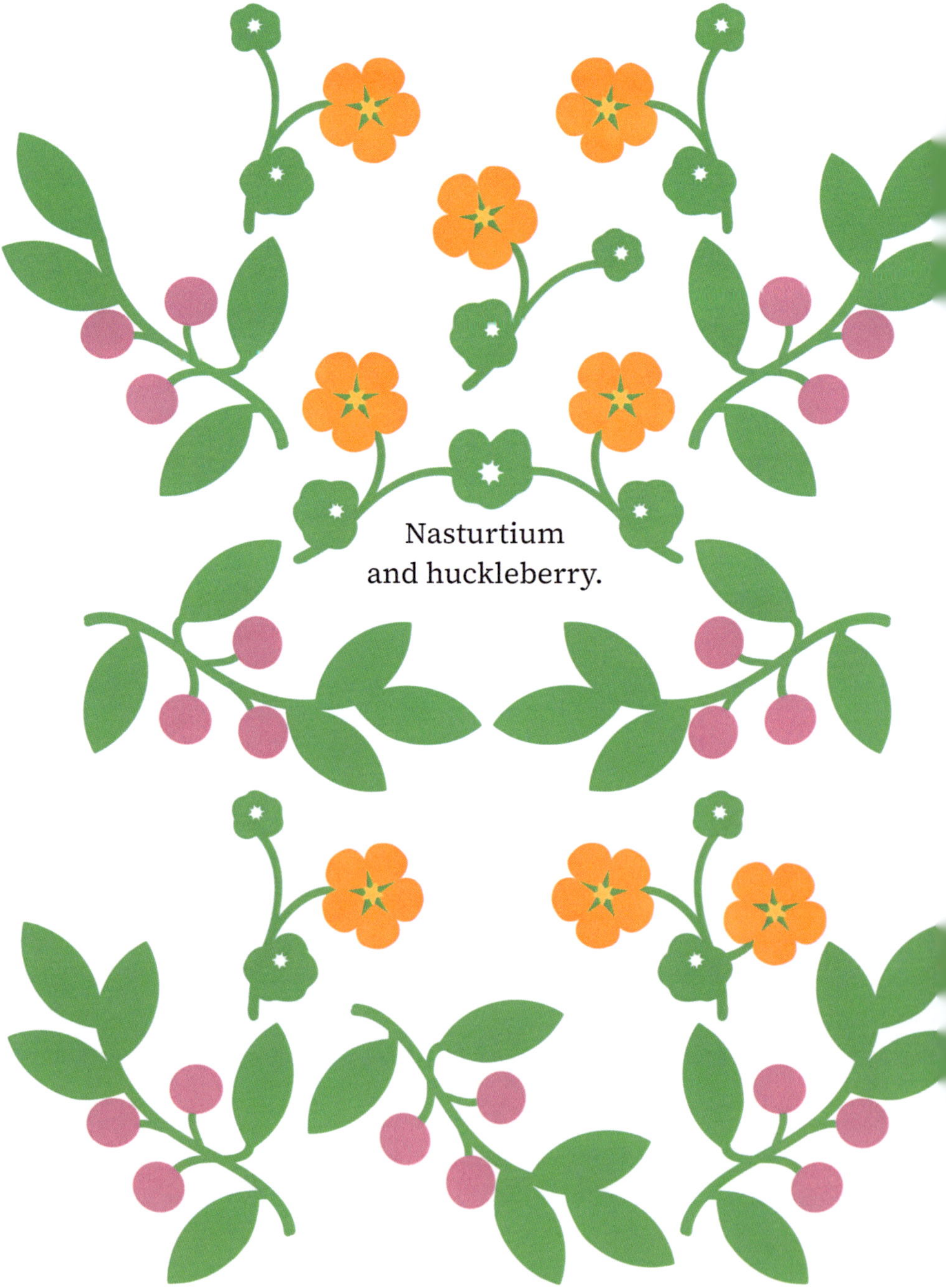

Nasturtium
and huckleberry.

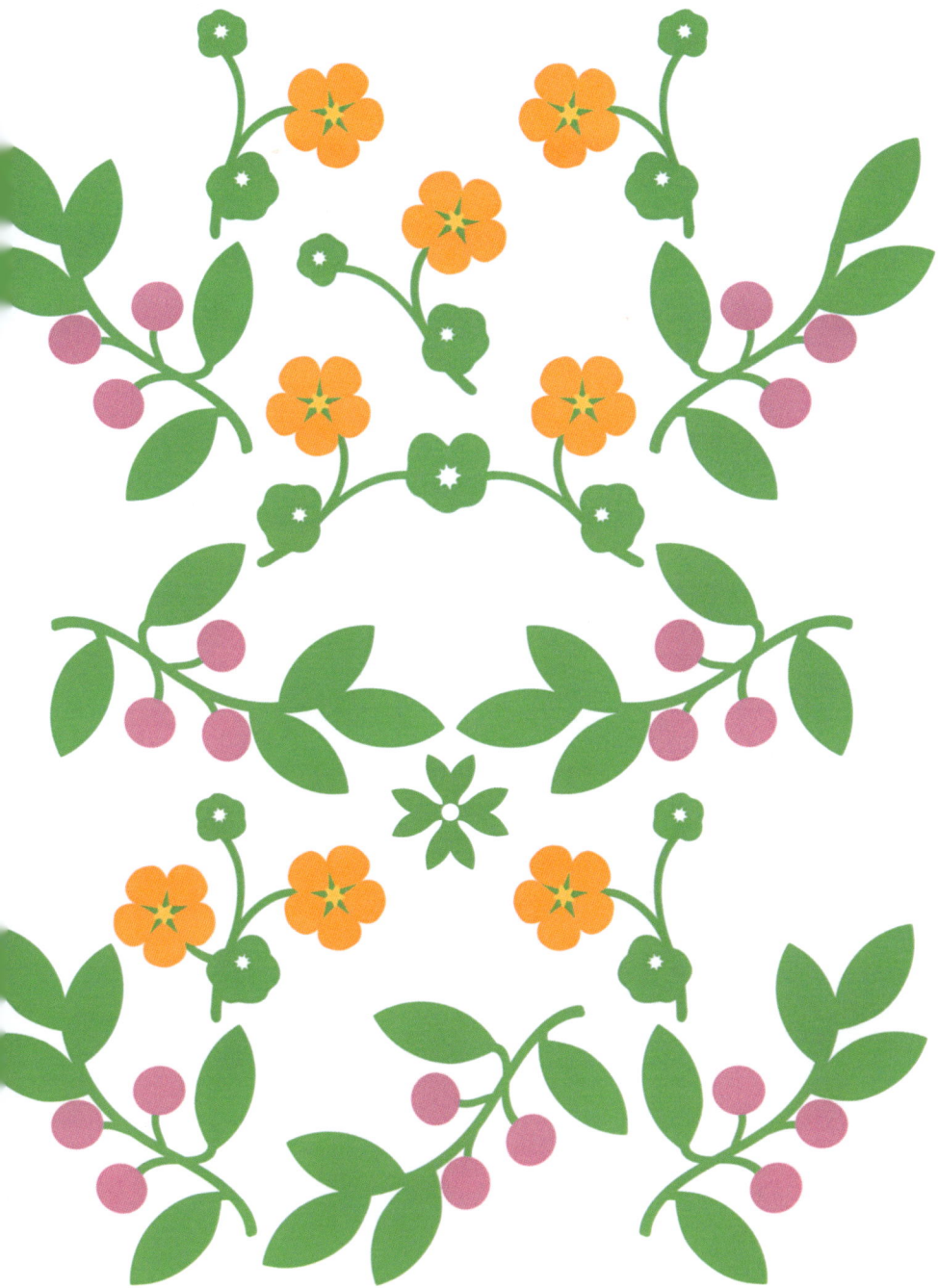

God's wondrous fruits are so rosy,
vibrant, dynamic, and pretty.

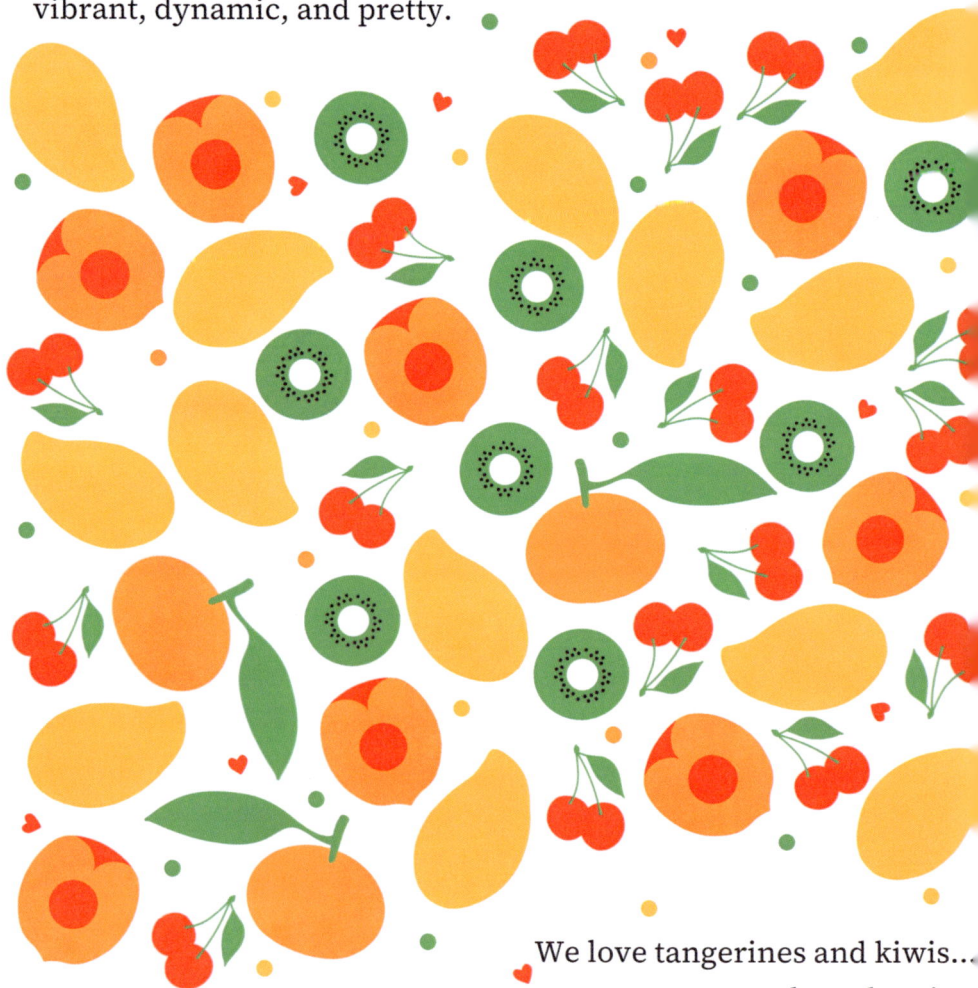

We love tangerines and kiwis...
mangos even more than cherries.
Peaches are true delicacies

But what's our favorite? Strawberries!

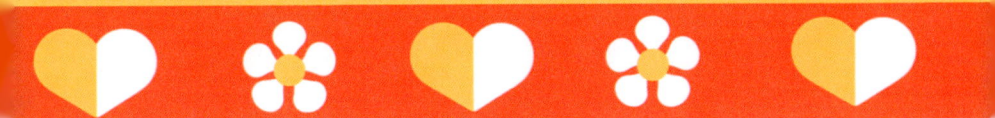

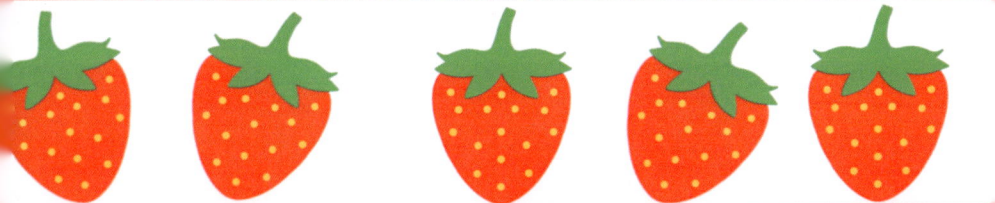

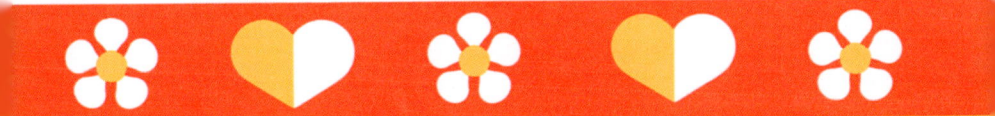

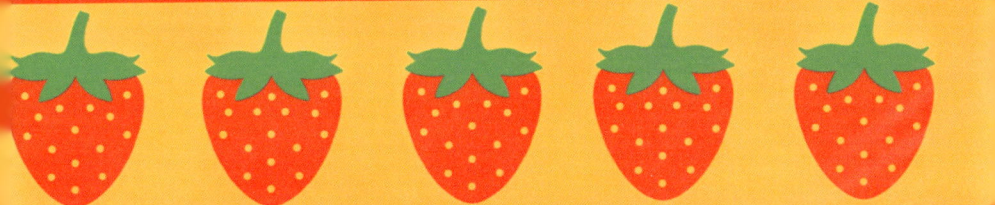

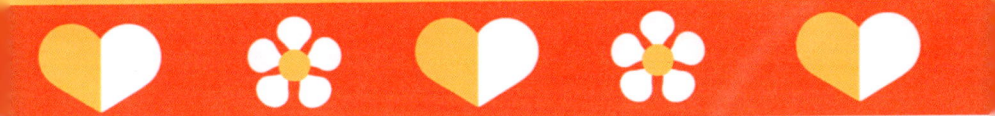

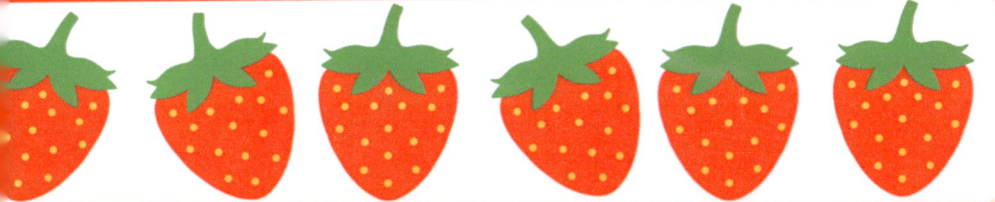

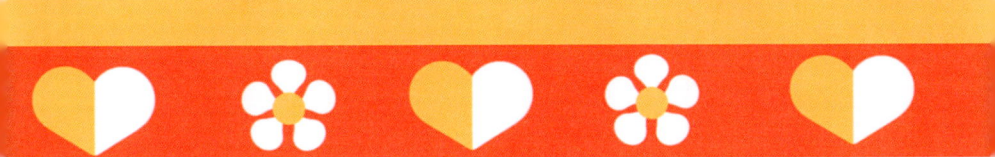

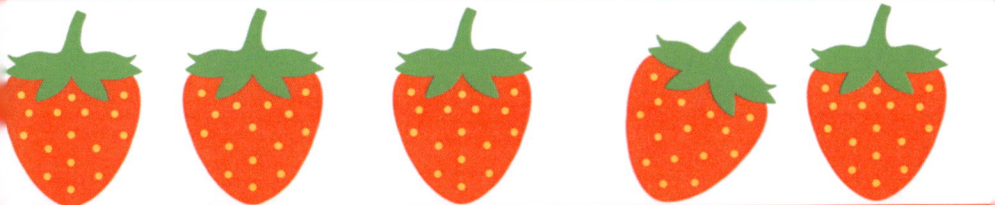

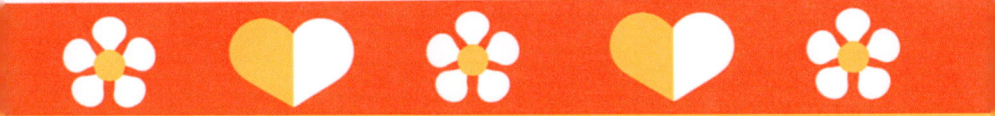

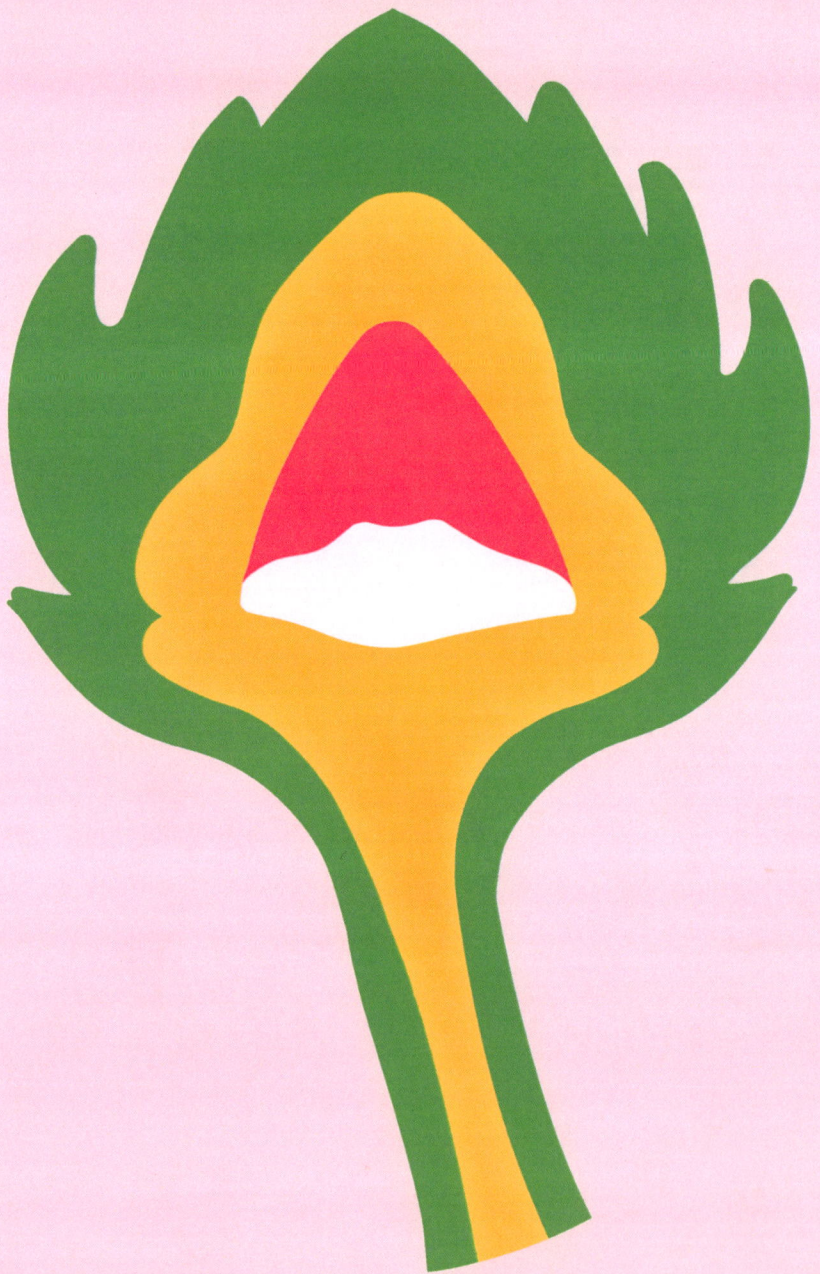

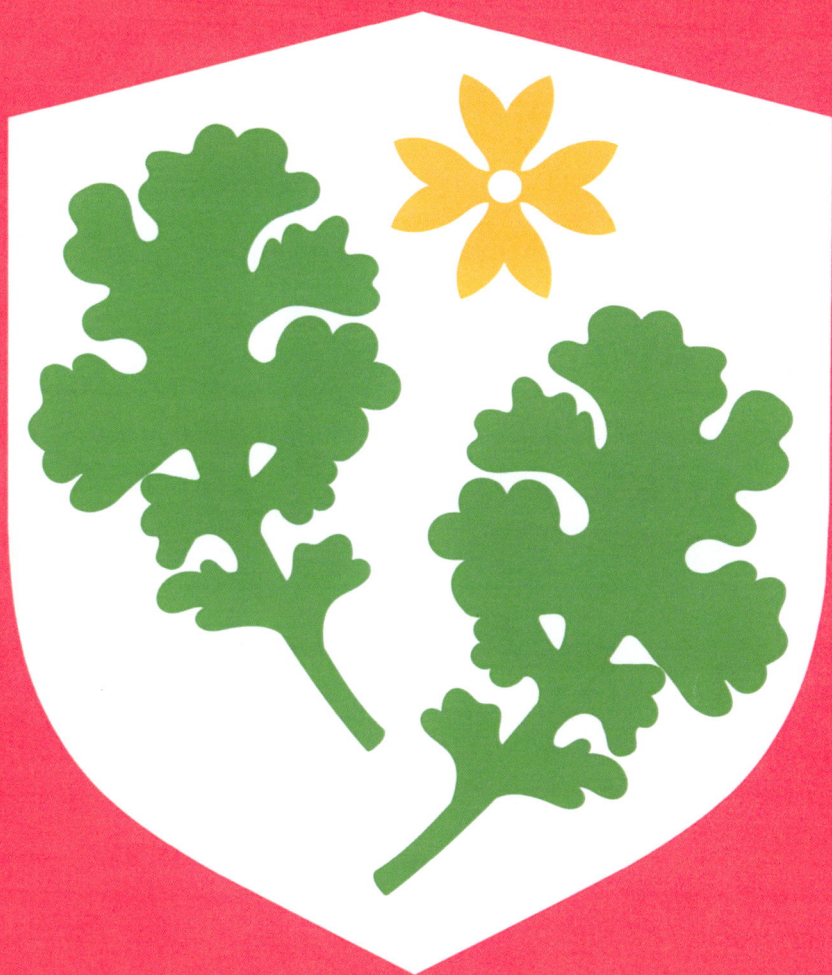

Vegetables are also wealthy.
Each one holds a full treasury.
They're rich in vitamins, you see,
proof of God's generosity.

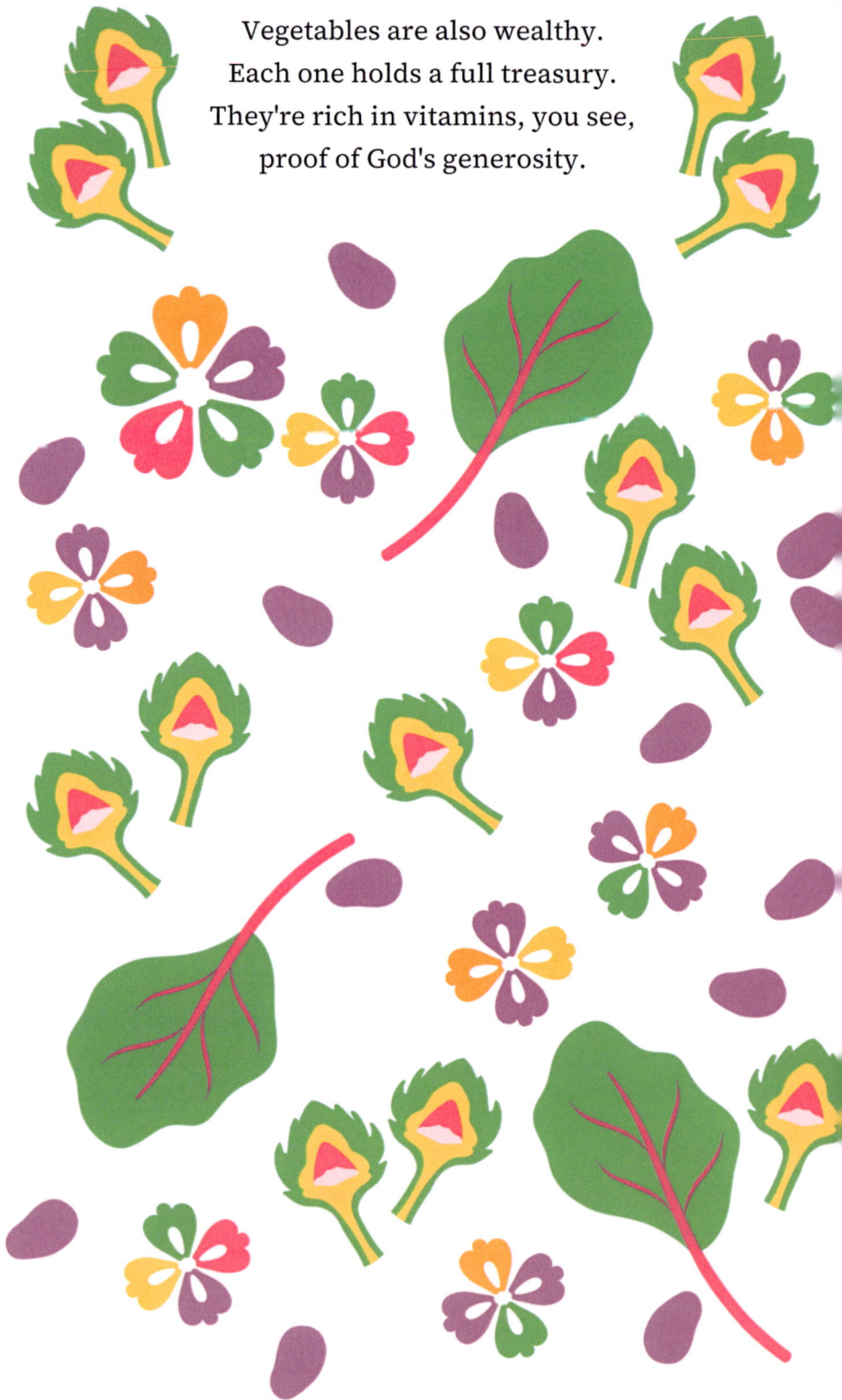

They all have healing properties
and nourish life remarkably.

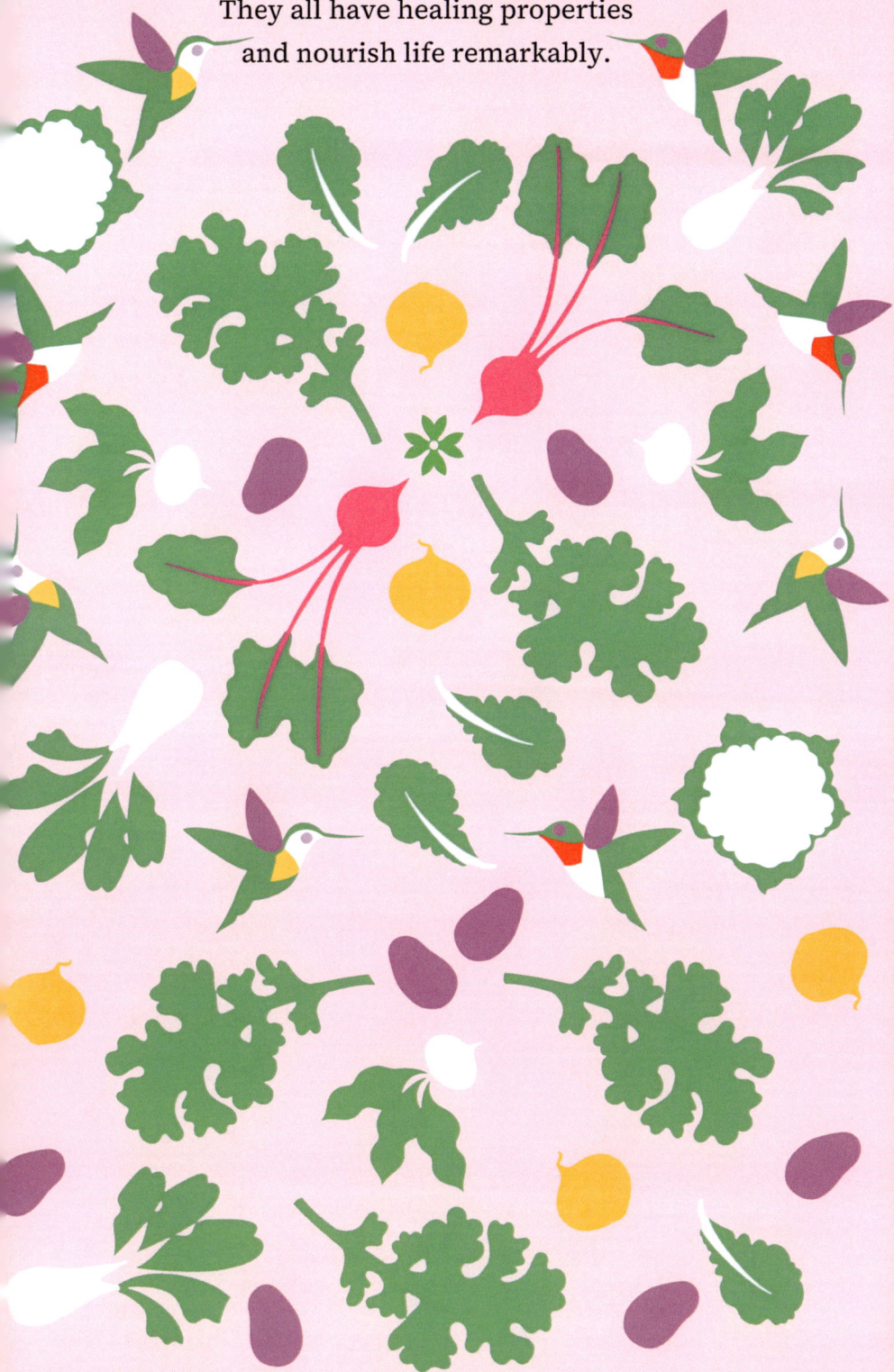

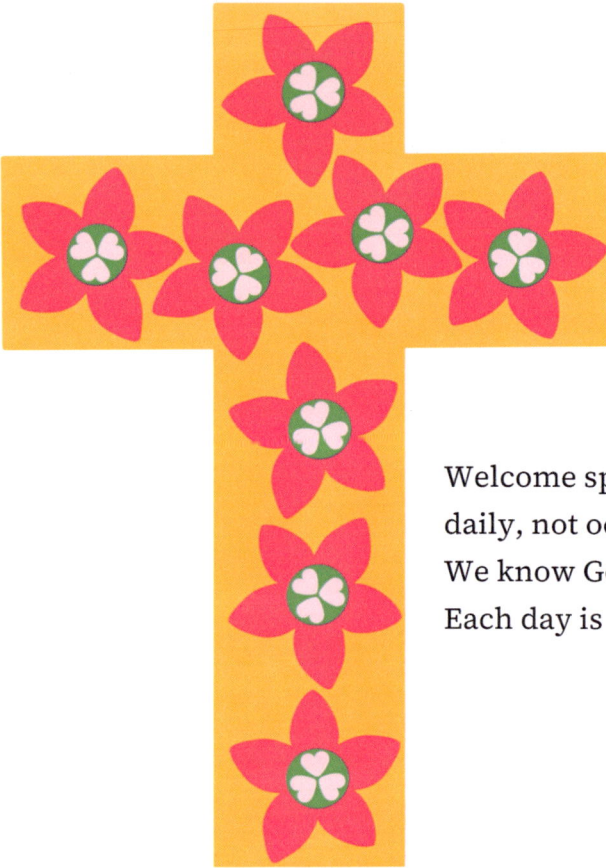

Welcome spirituality,
daily, not occasionally.
We know God works amazingly.
Each day is made just perfectly.

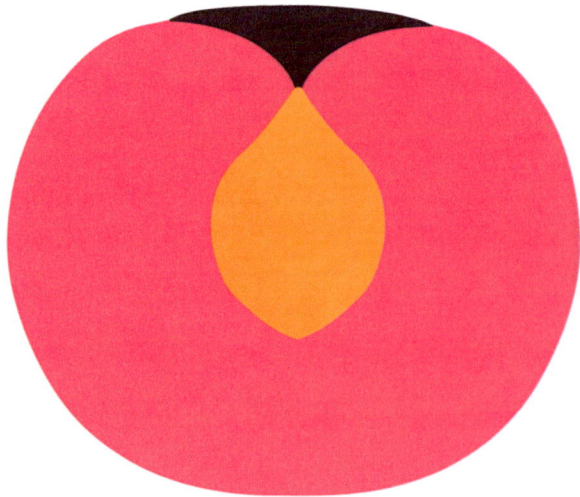

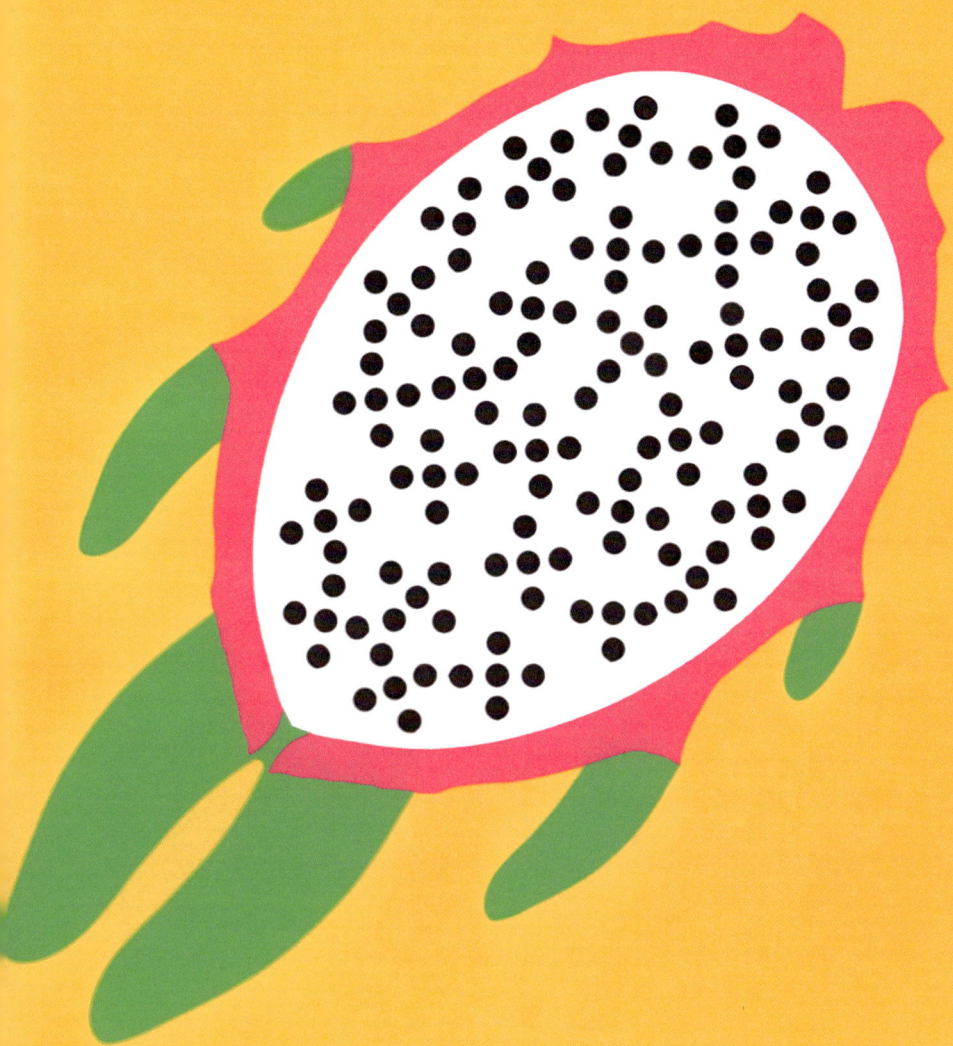

Even if you are a foodie,
or have been described as picky,

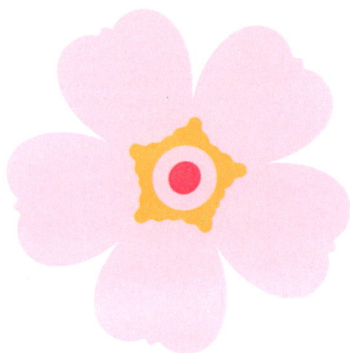

nevertheless, you must agree:
there is a prized variety
of edible flowers and seeds.

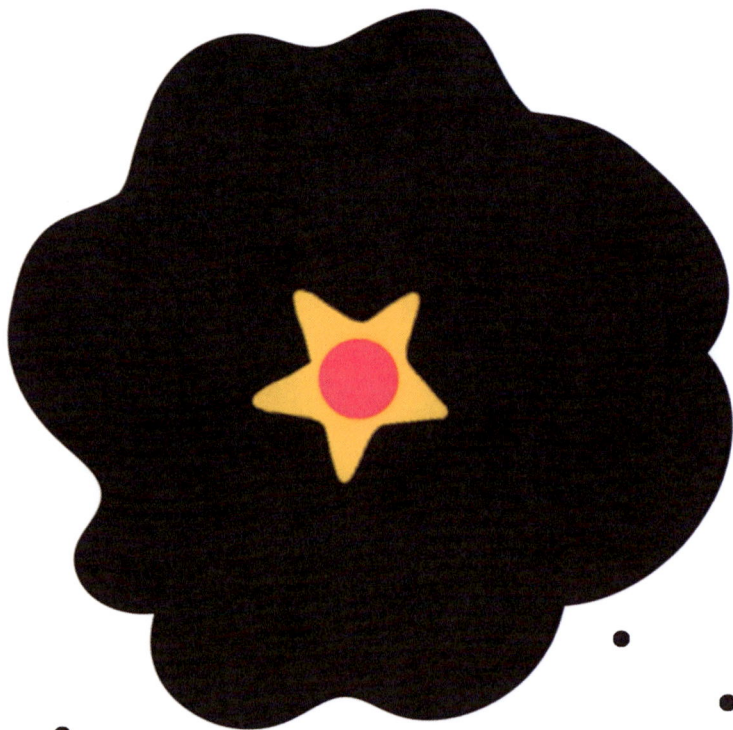

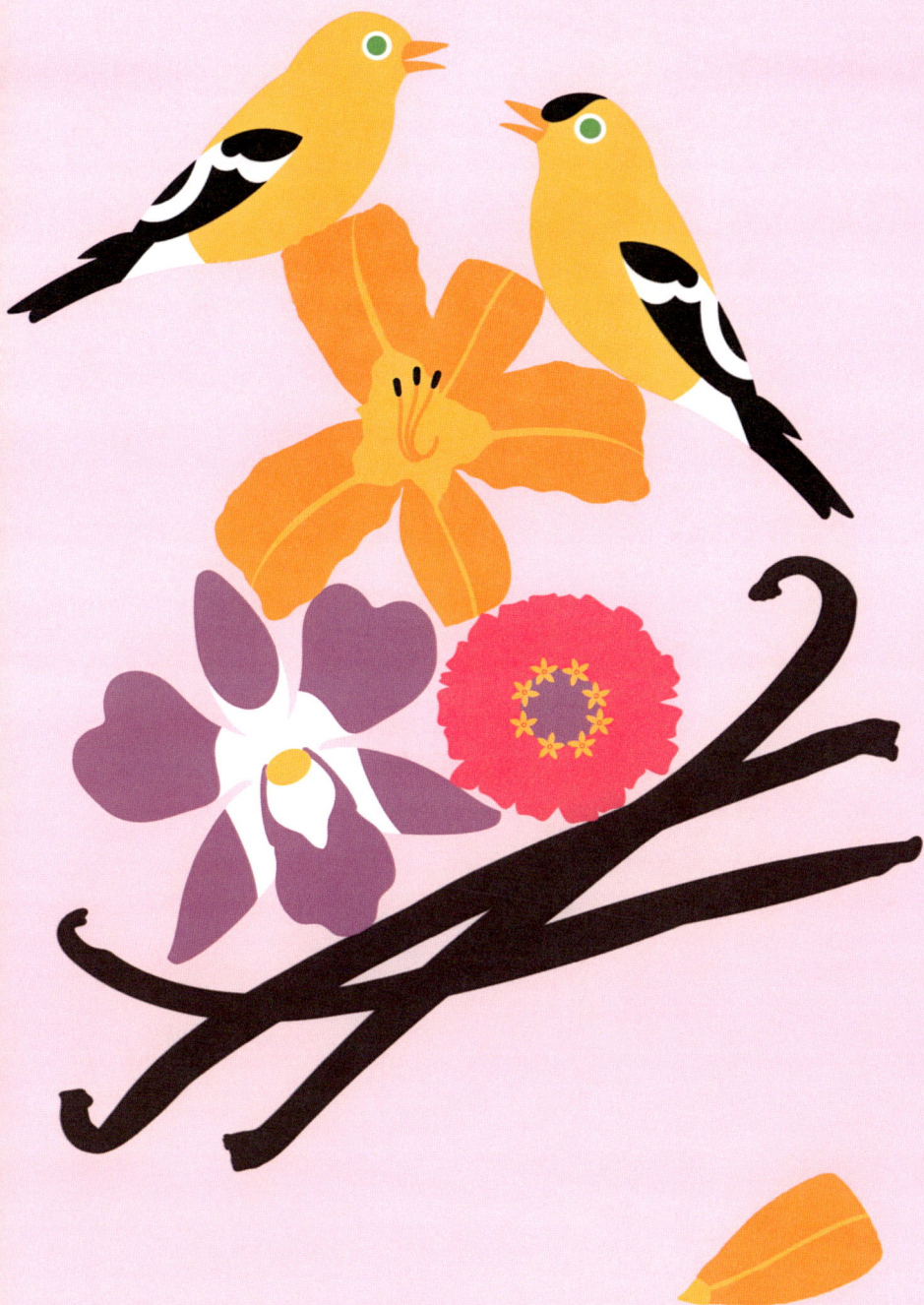

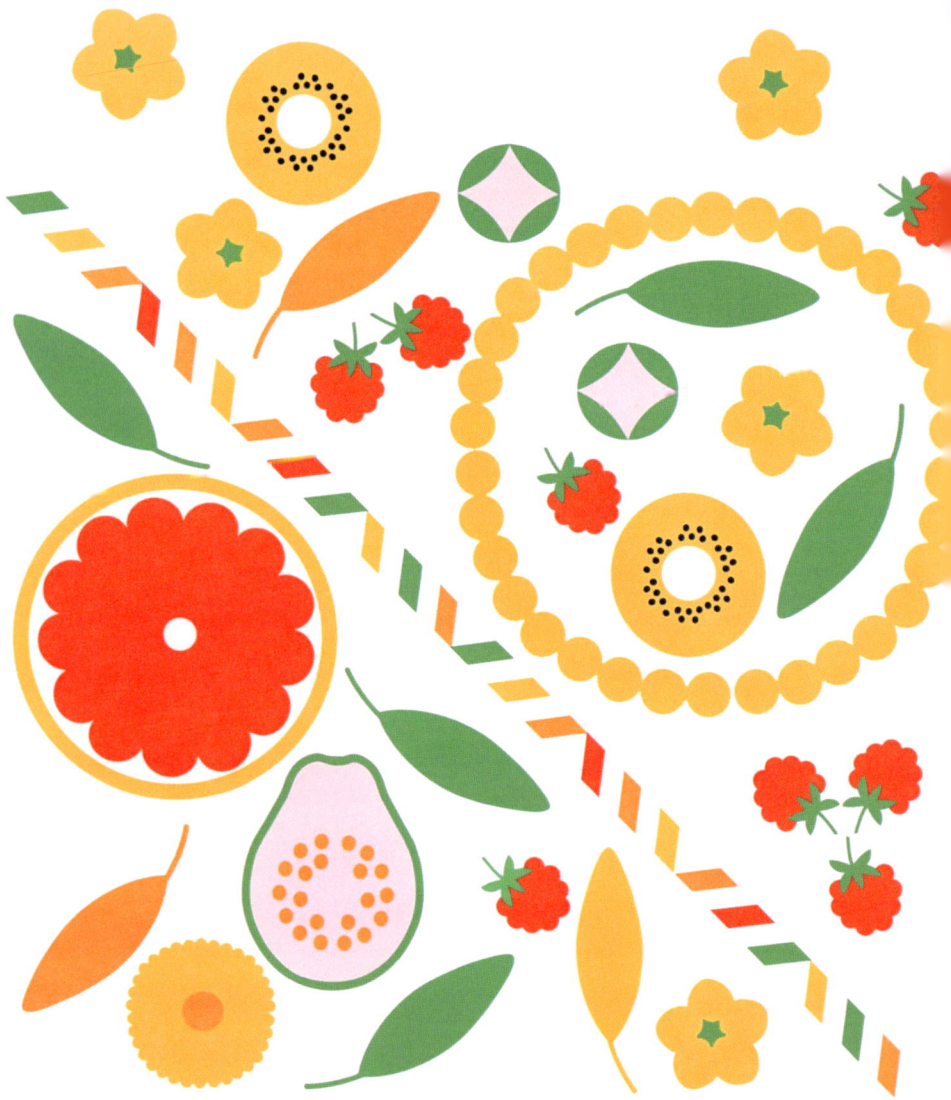

God clothes the earth so carefully,
with food growing beautifully.

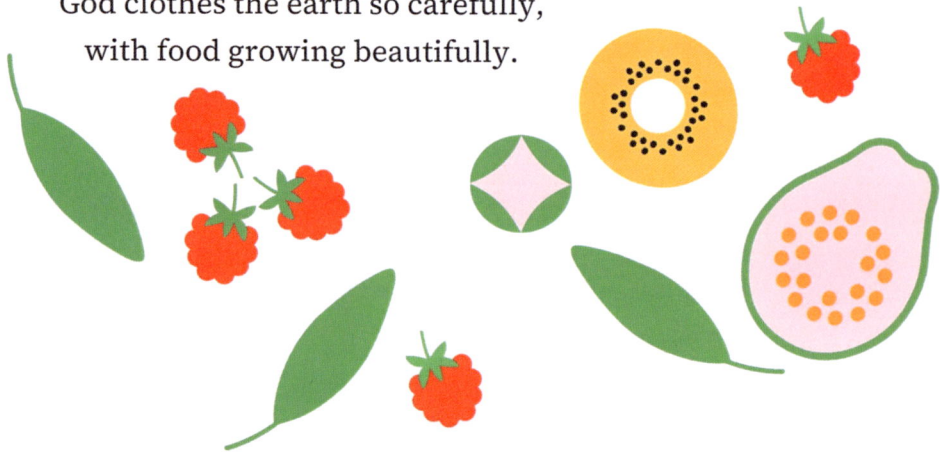

So, choose farms over factories.
Buy sweet fruit instead of candies.

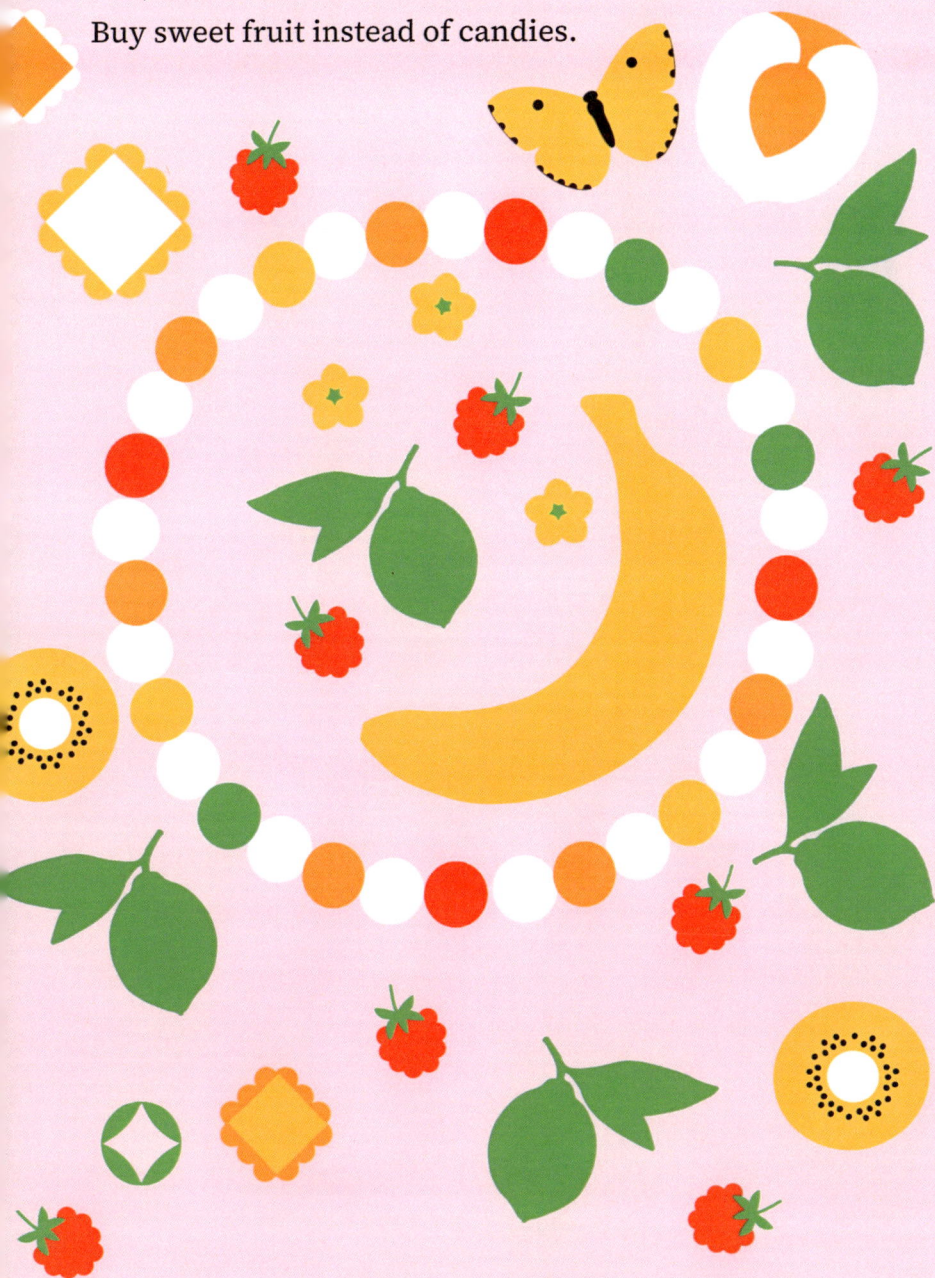

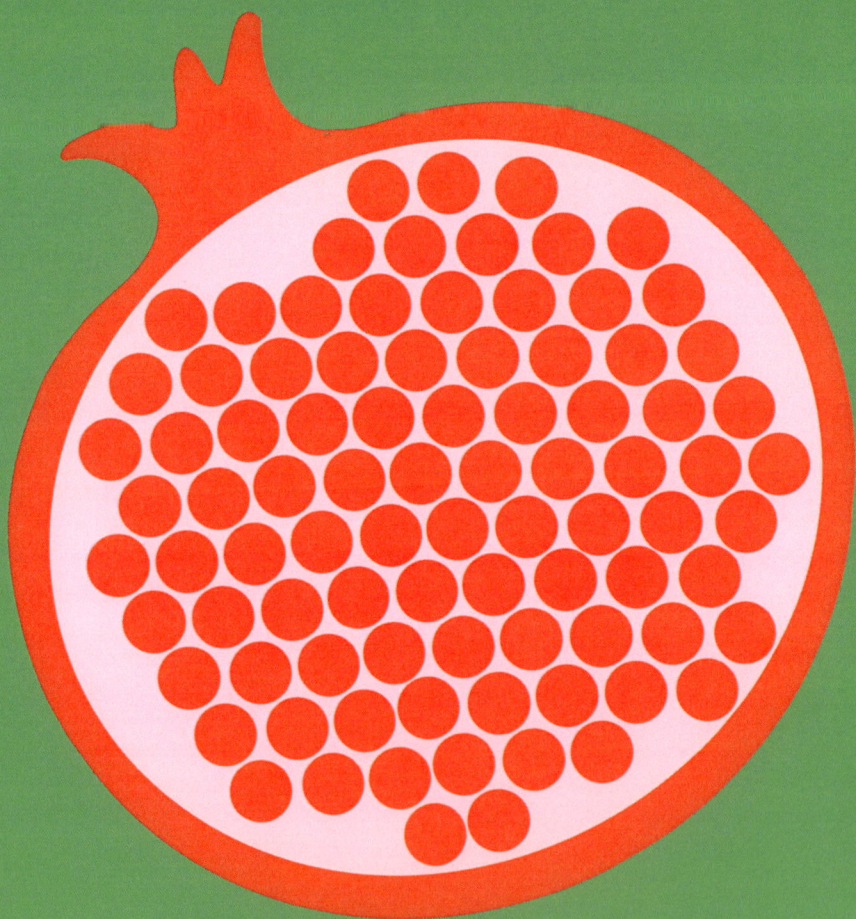

Making choices can be tricky,
when packaging is quite witty.
Avoid the empty calories.
Eat real food quite happily.

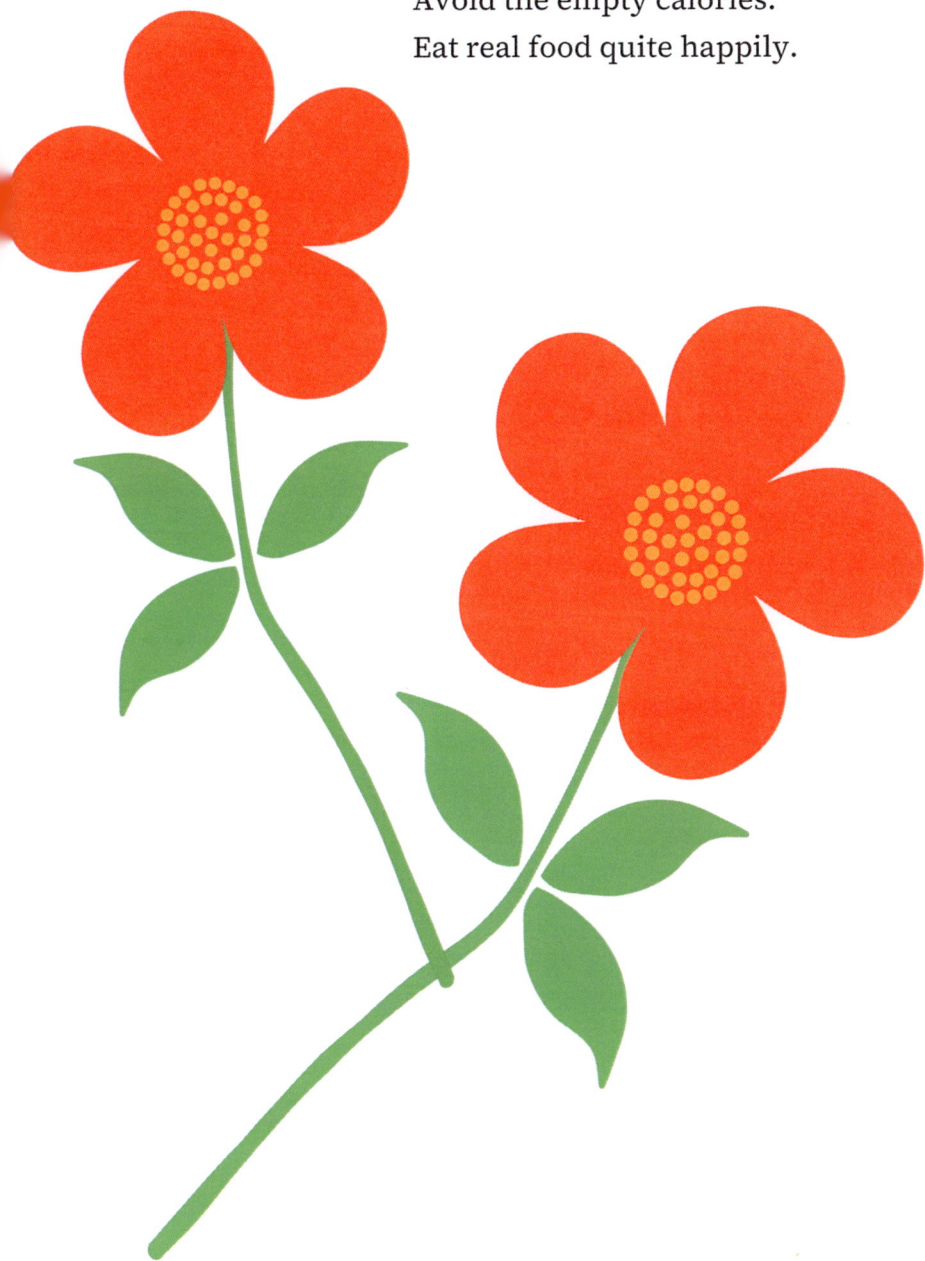

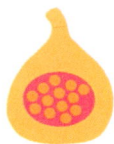

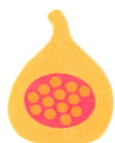

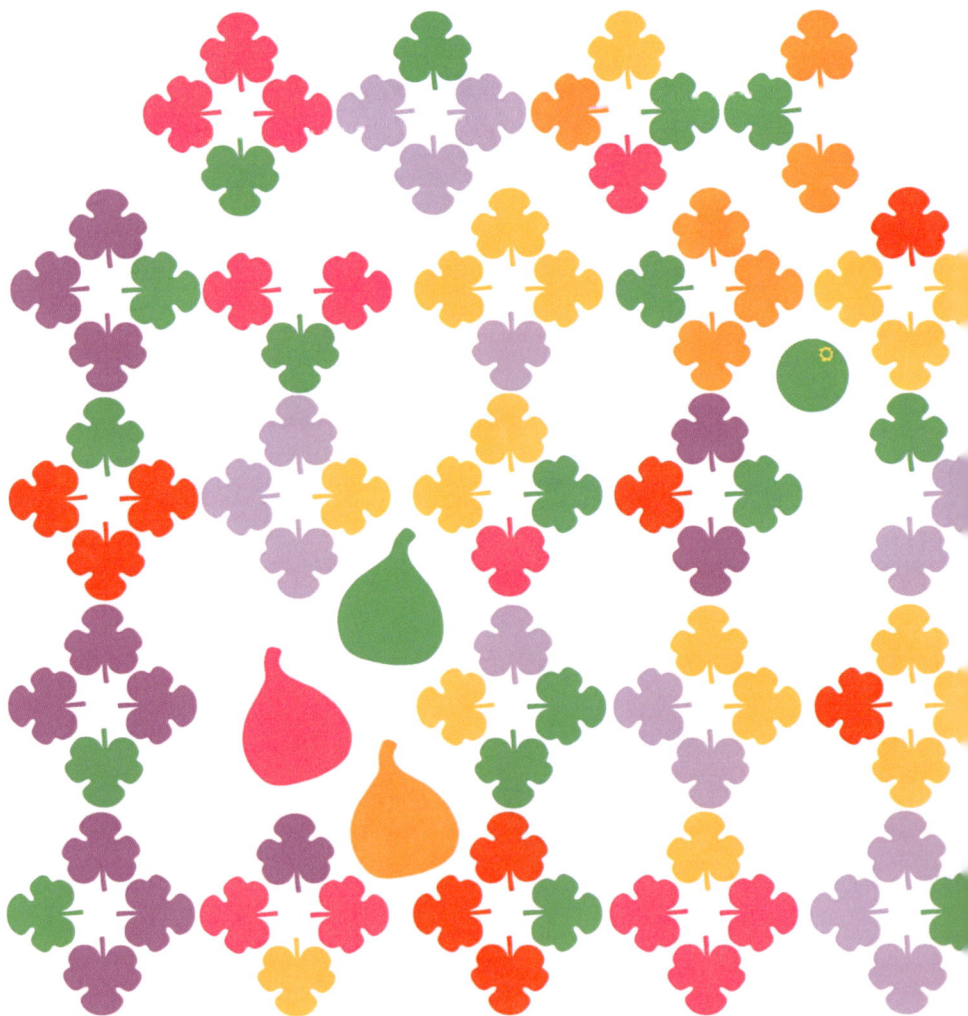

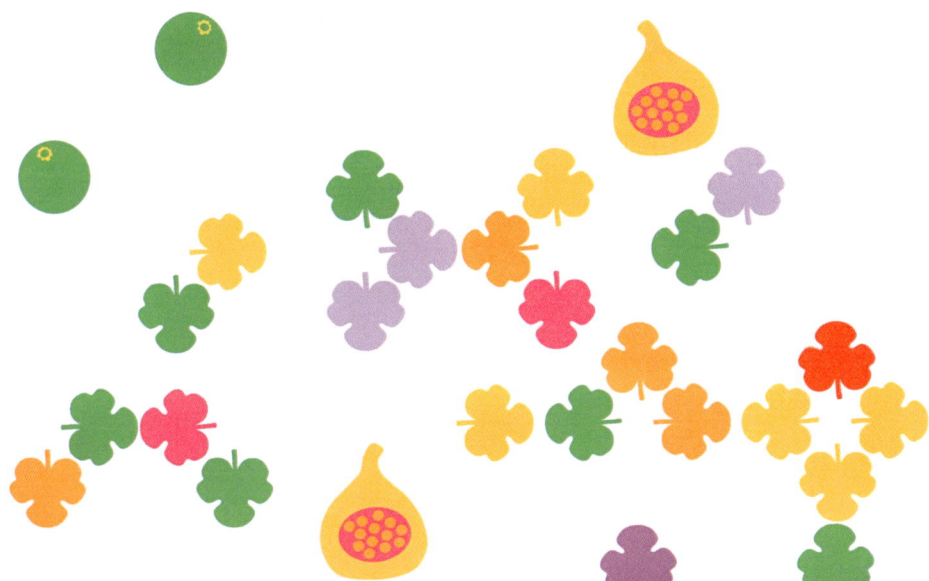

Select figs or amla berries,
less junk food, more fresh groceries.

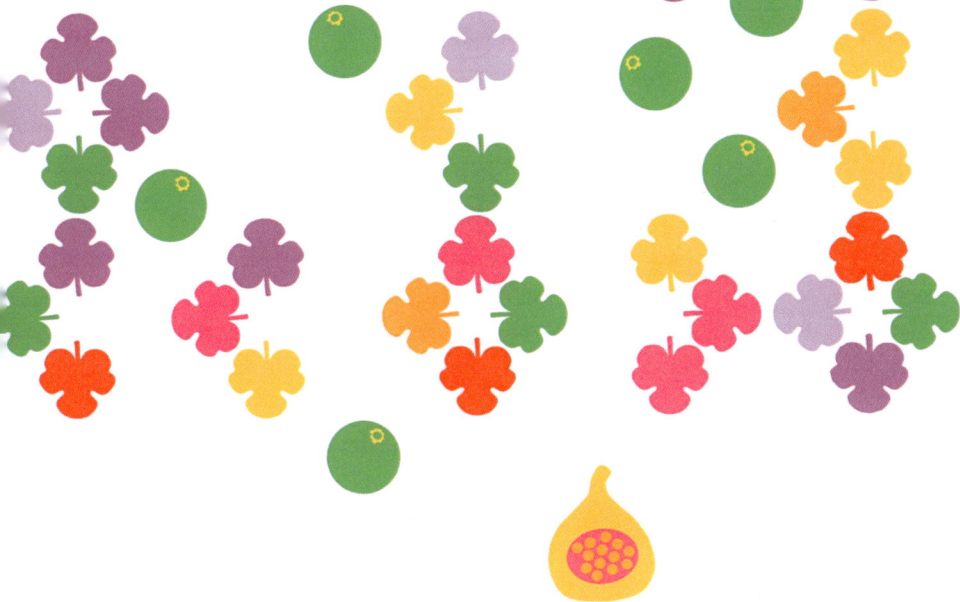

Heirloom seeds are truly holy.
Without them, no garden party.

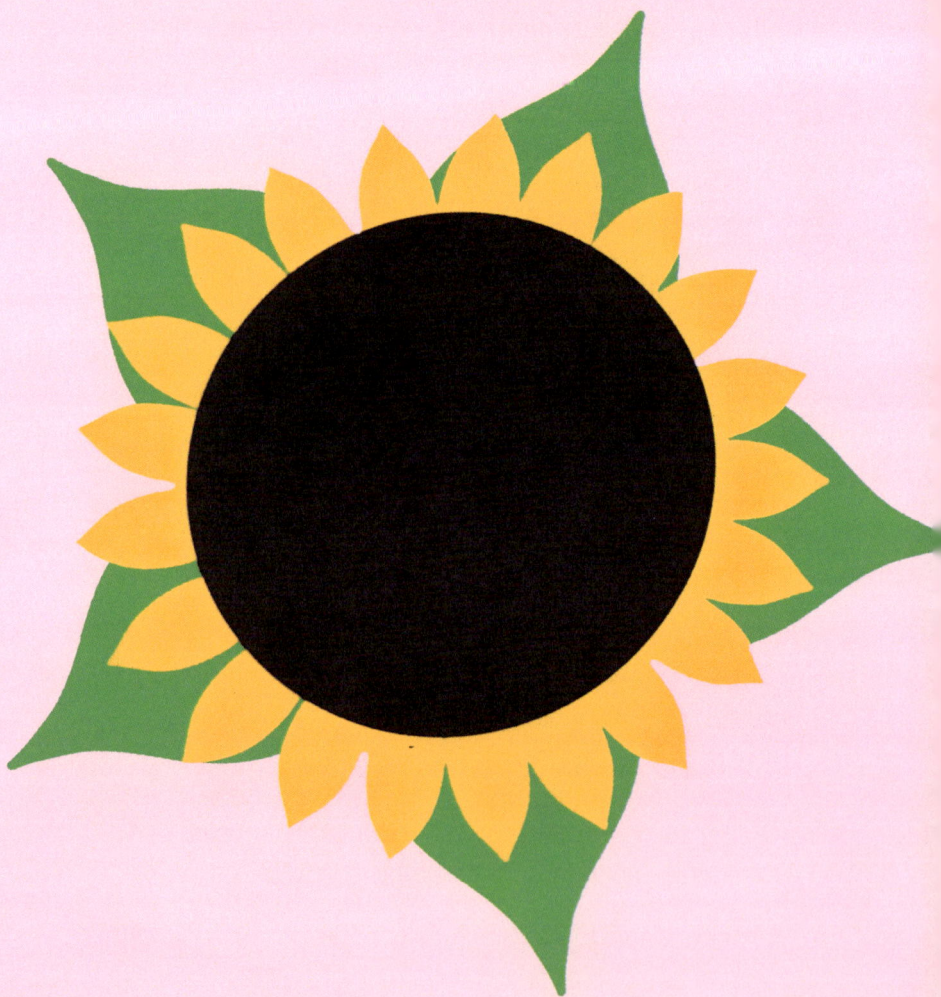

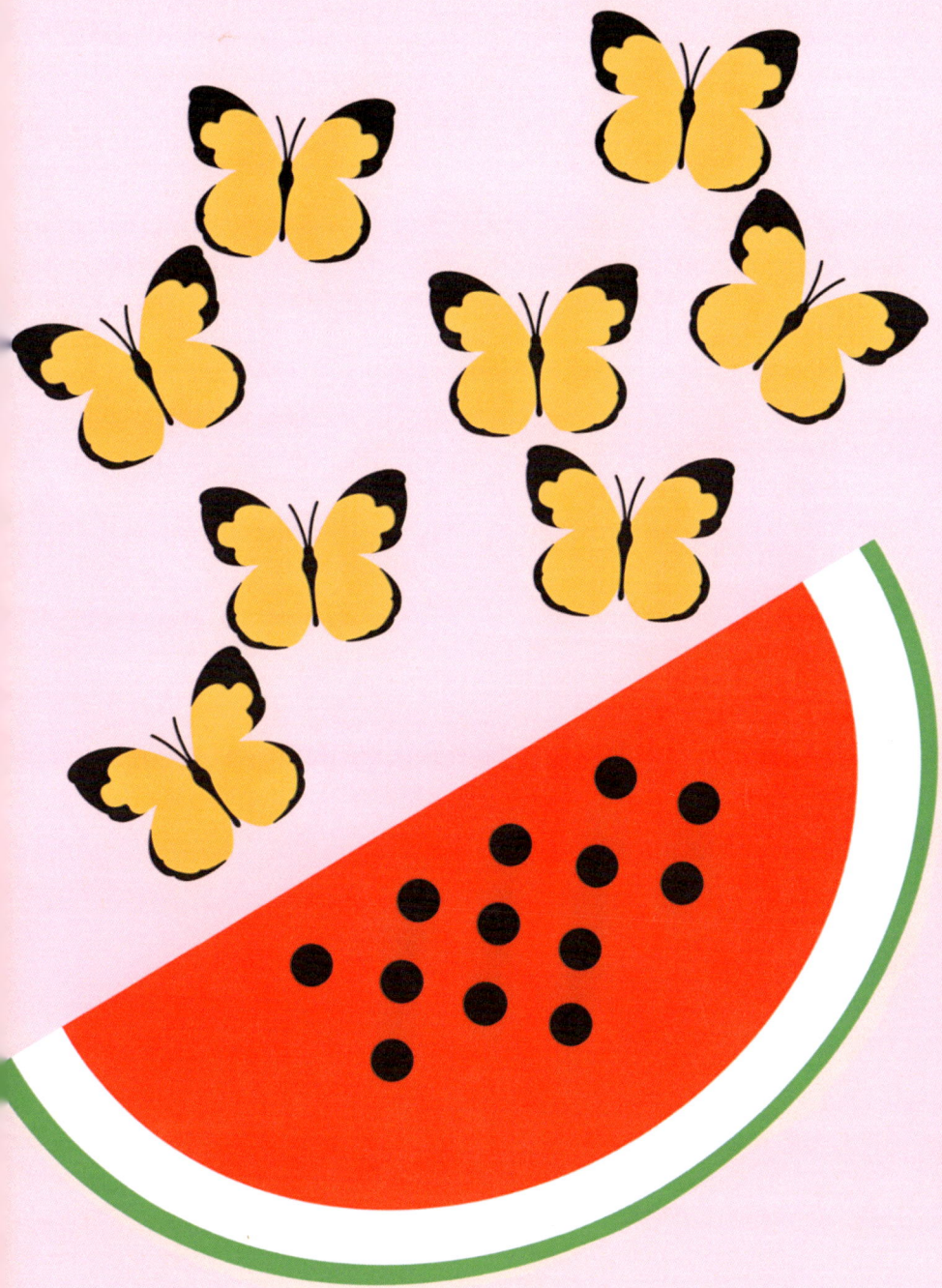

Plants give us all that energy.
Let us offer thanks sincerely,
for food enjoyed, especially…
for beans, which are high qualit
great for protein, and are heart

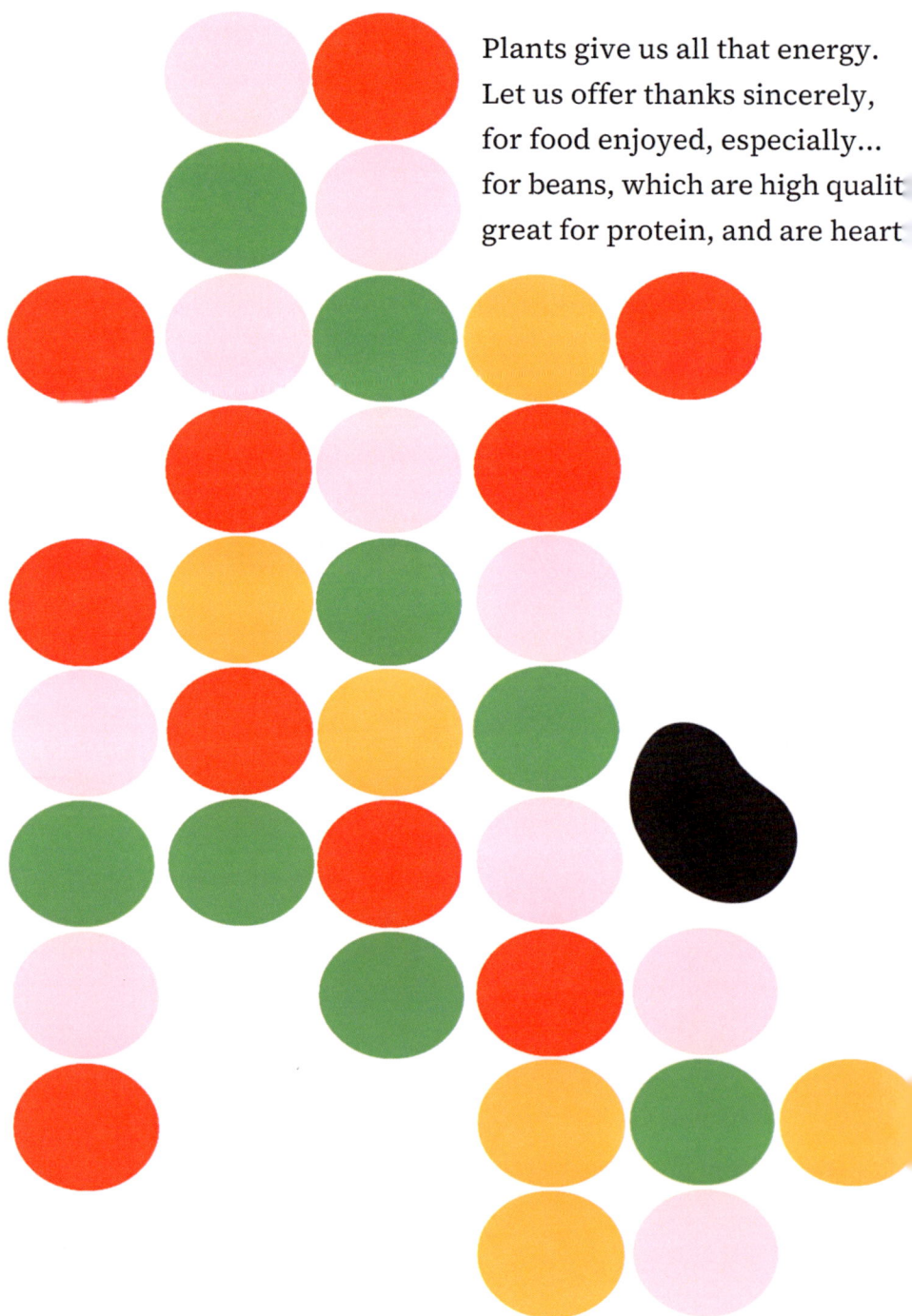

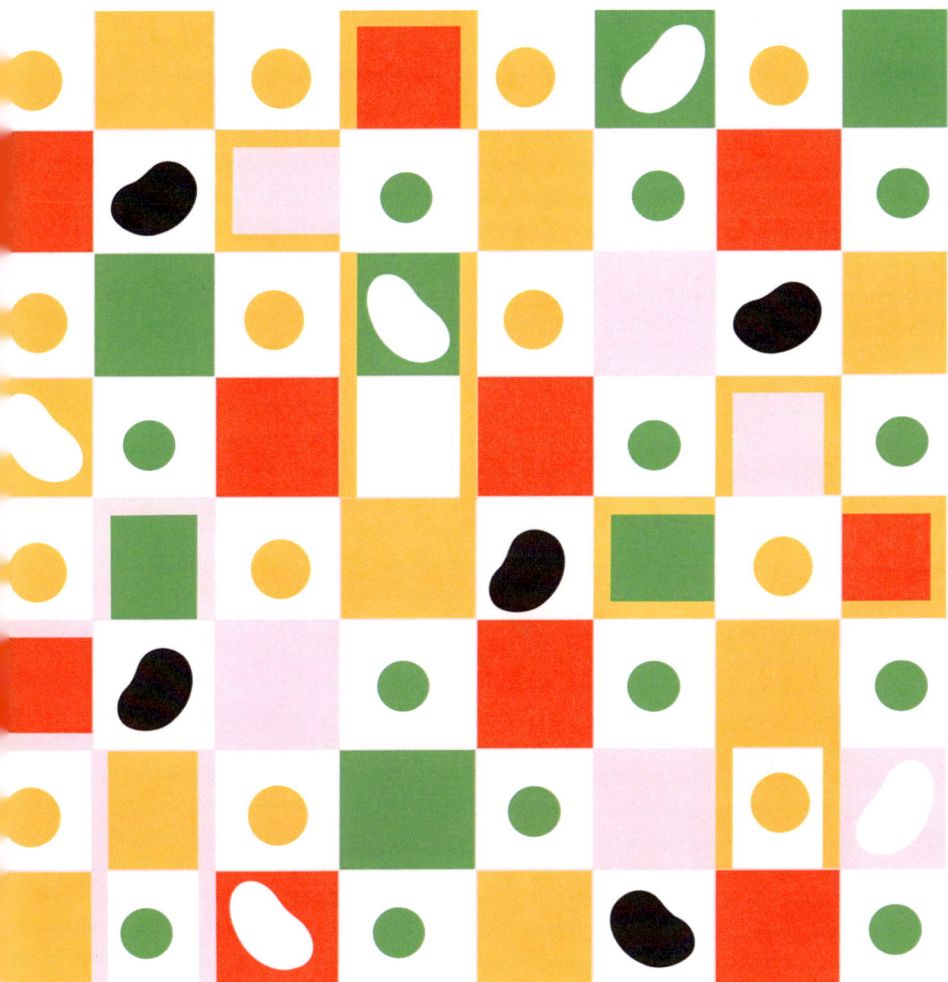

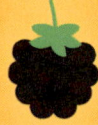

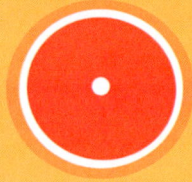

Support organic farming, please.
Our vines, bushes, and of course trees,
should always be pesticide-free.
Help the planet, save bumblebees.

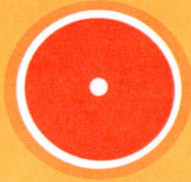

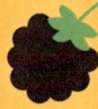

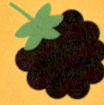

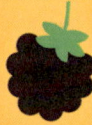

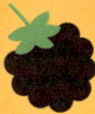

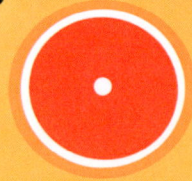

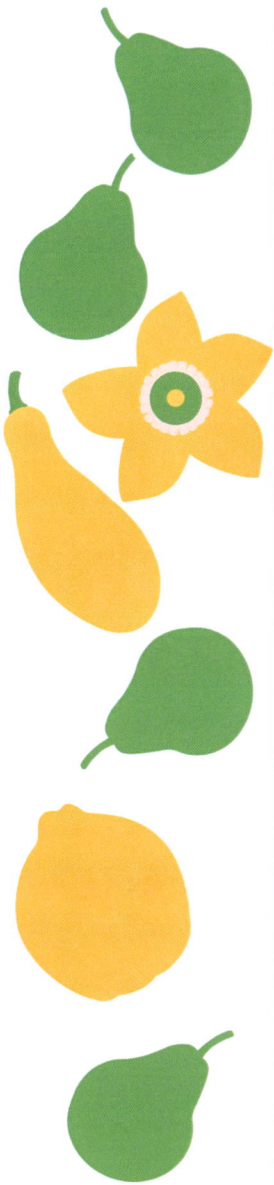

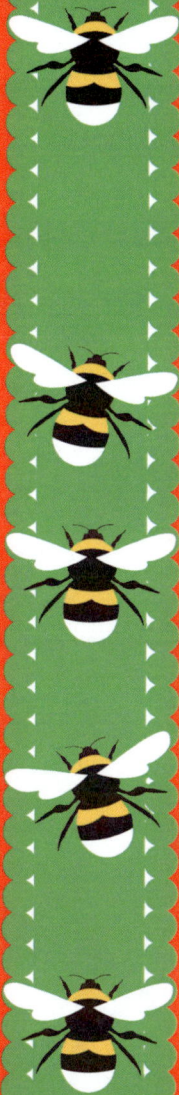

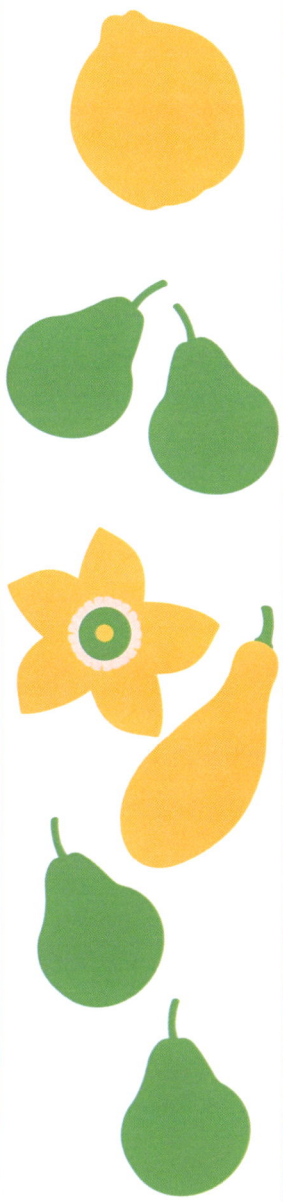

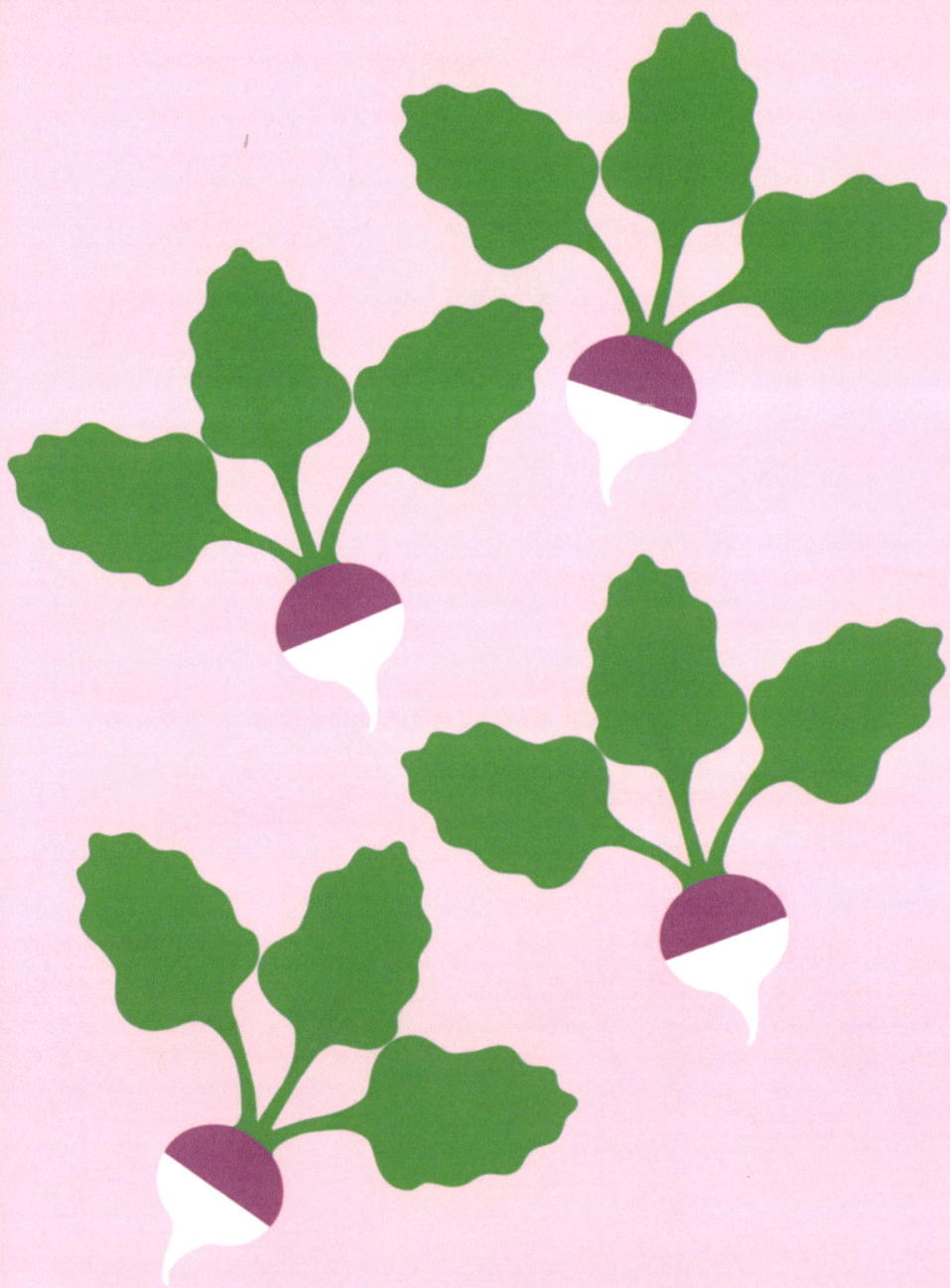

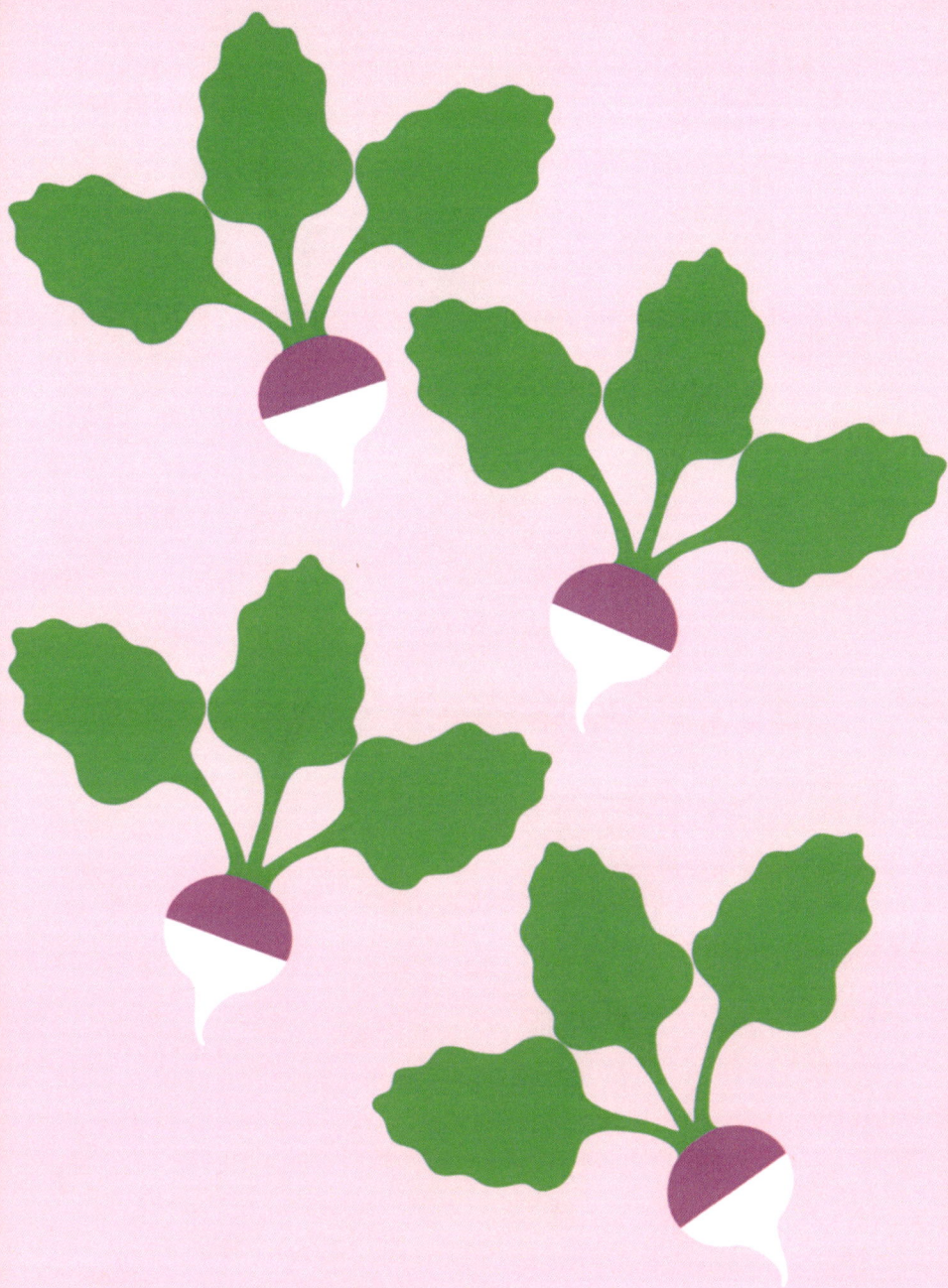

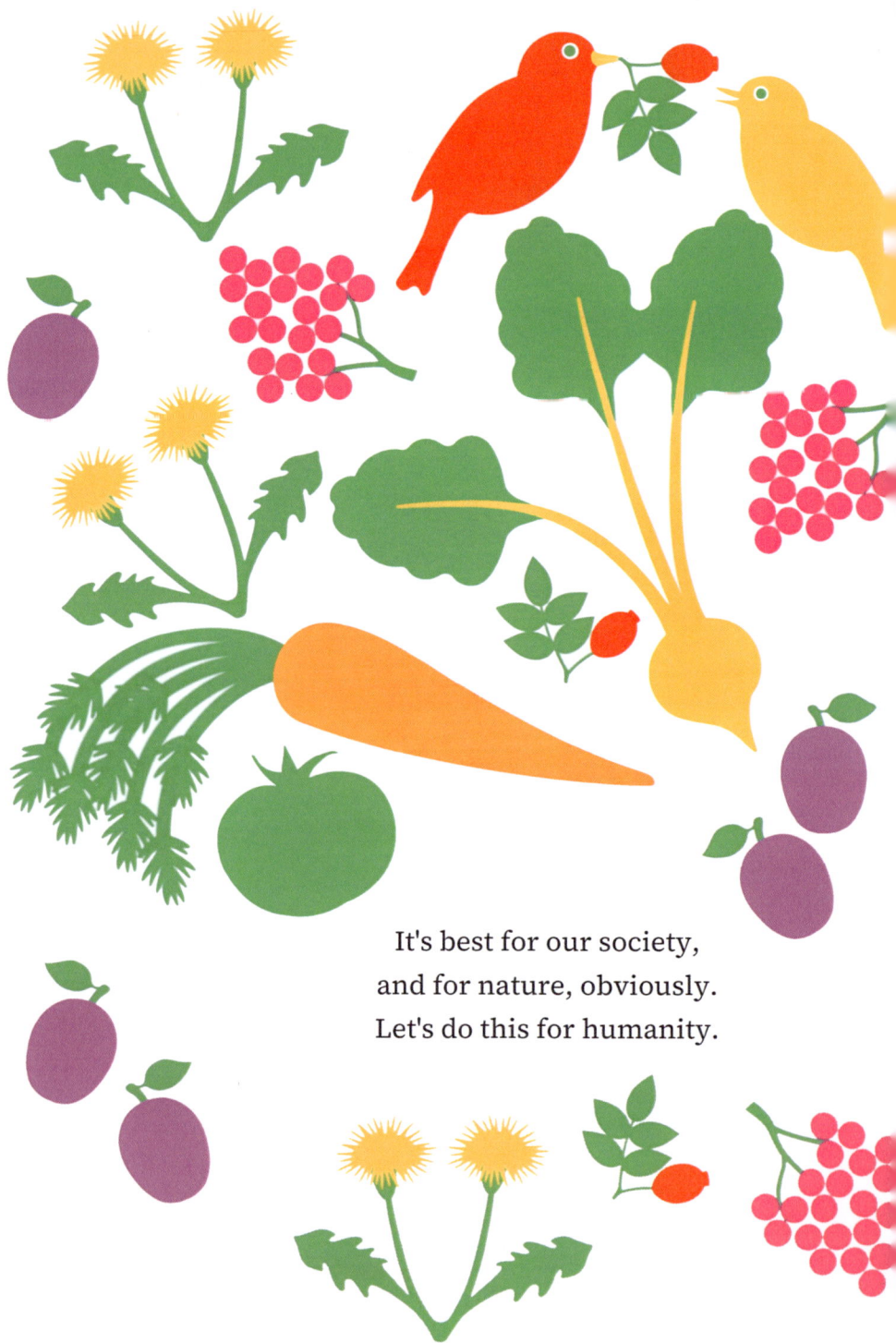

It's best for our society,
and for nature, obviously.
Let's do this for humanity.

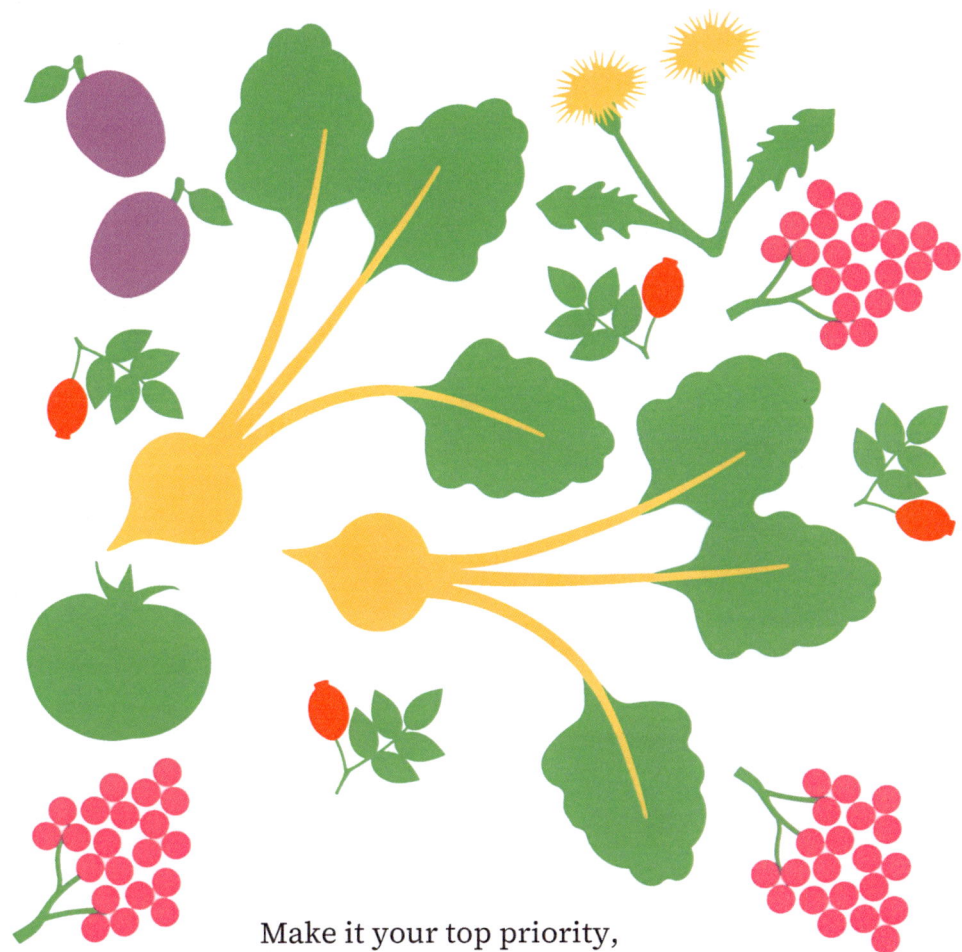

Make it your top priority,
to do what's right. Act consciously.
Eating vegetables is the key!
And look for food grown locally.

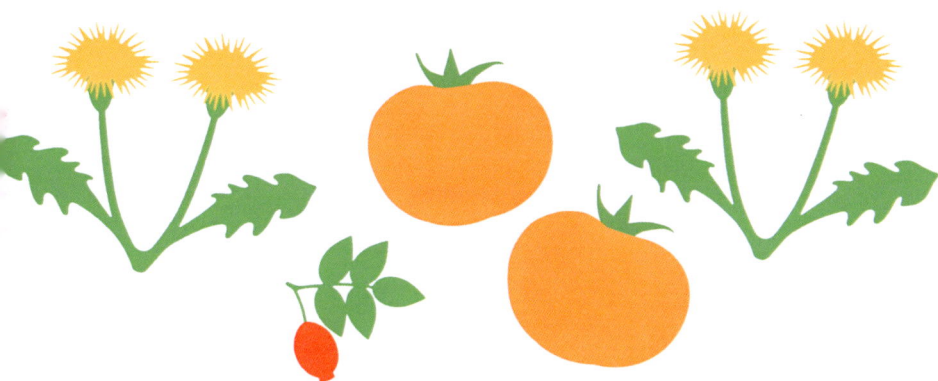

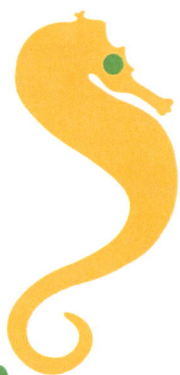

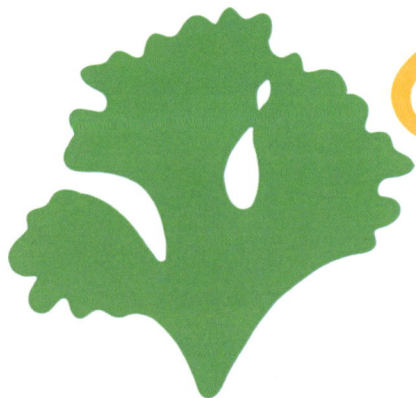

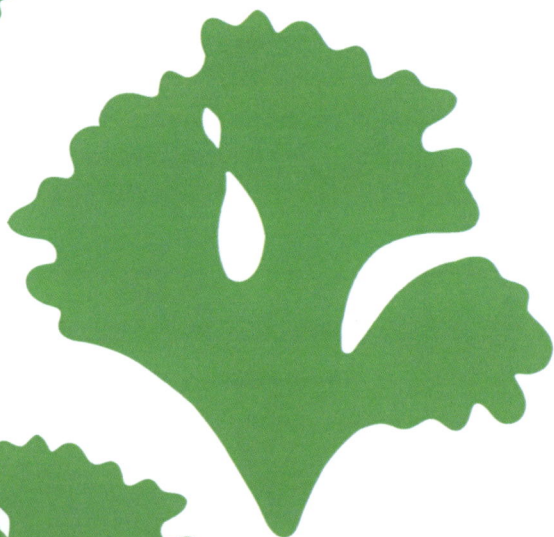

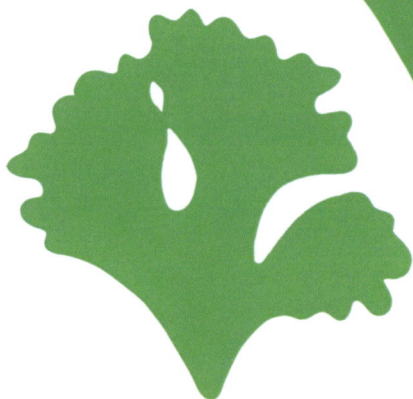

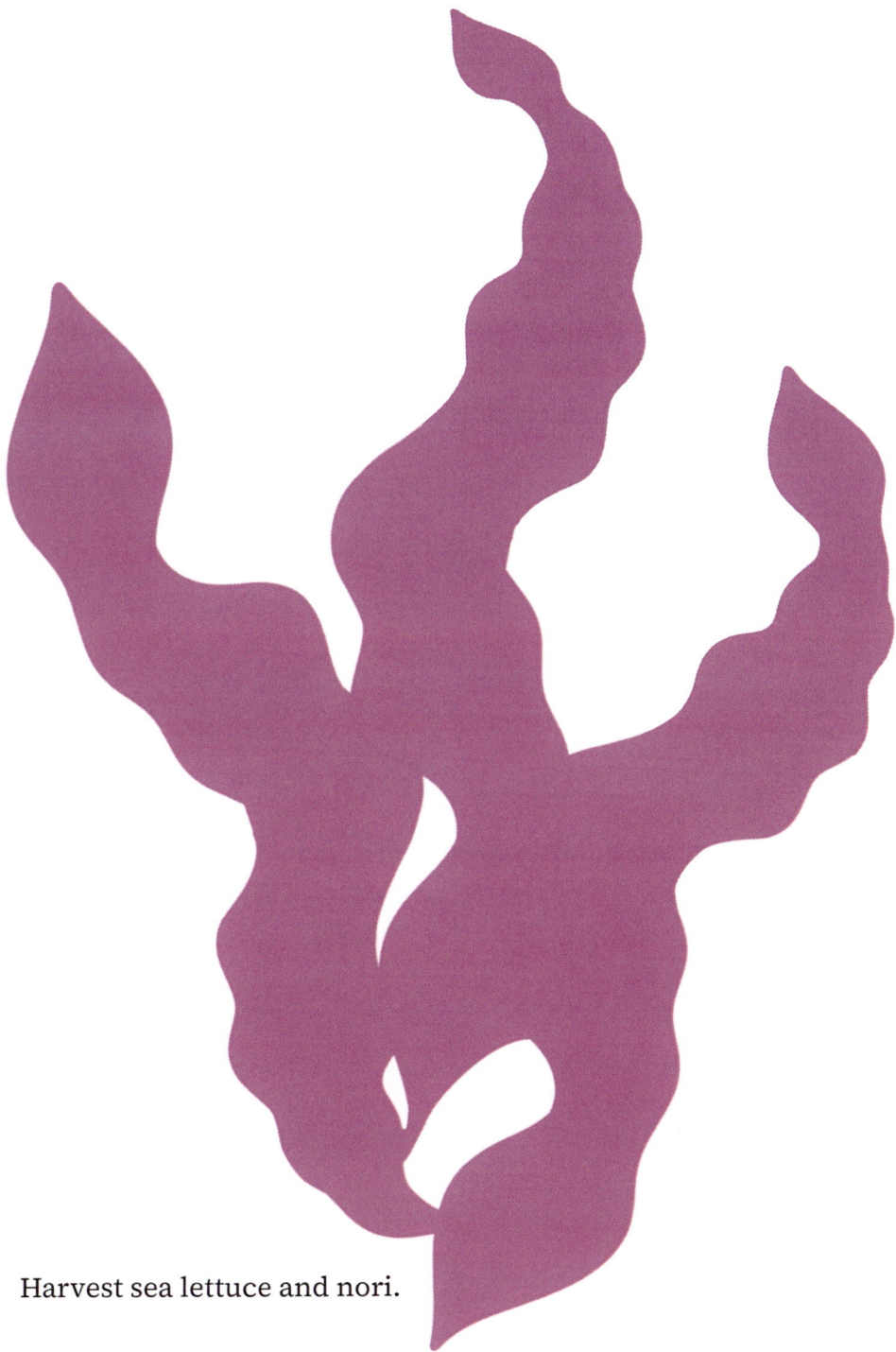

Harvest sea lettuce and nori.

Go green with your community.

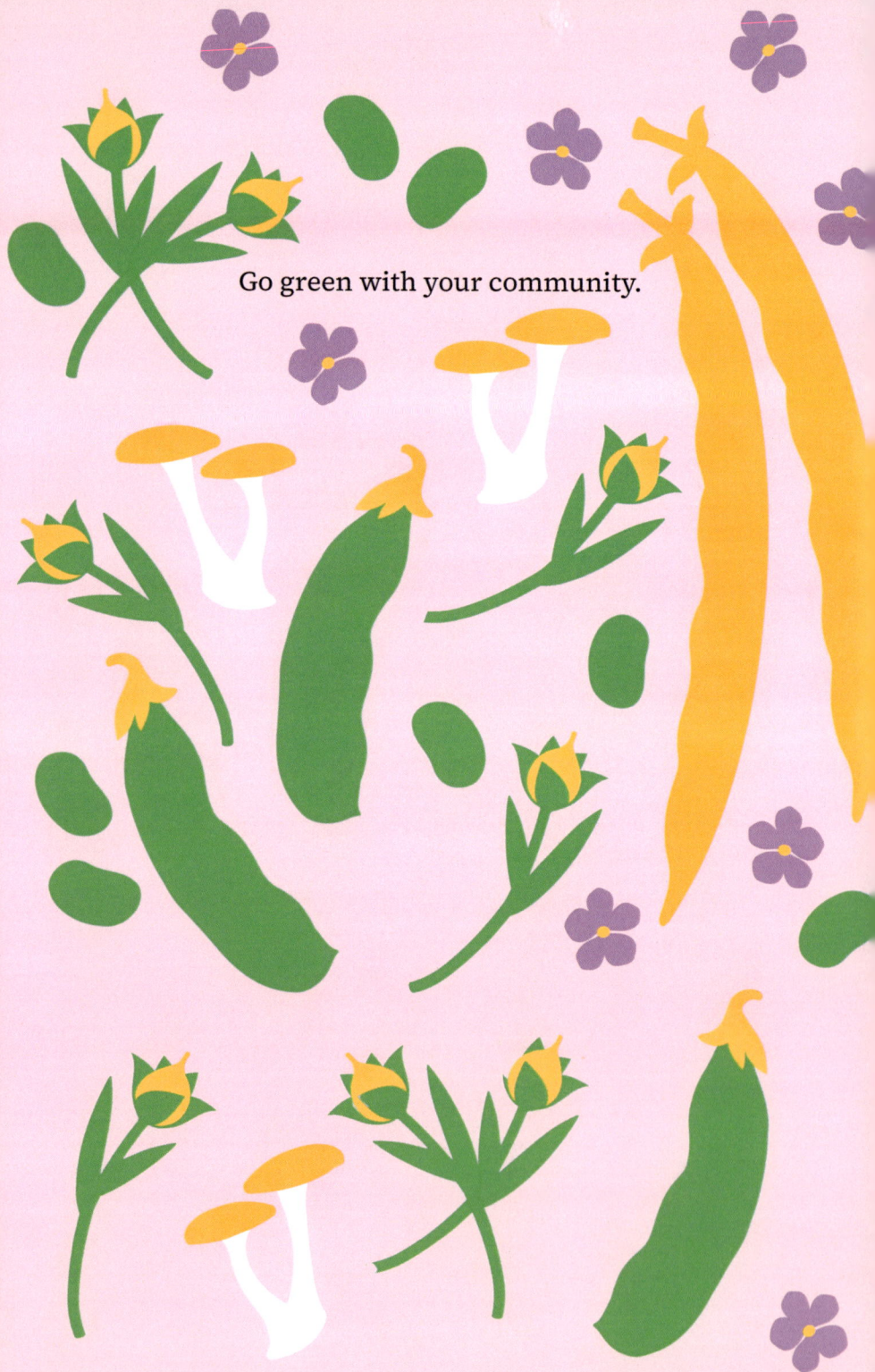

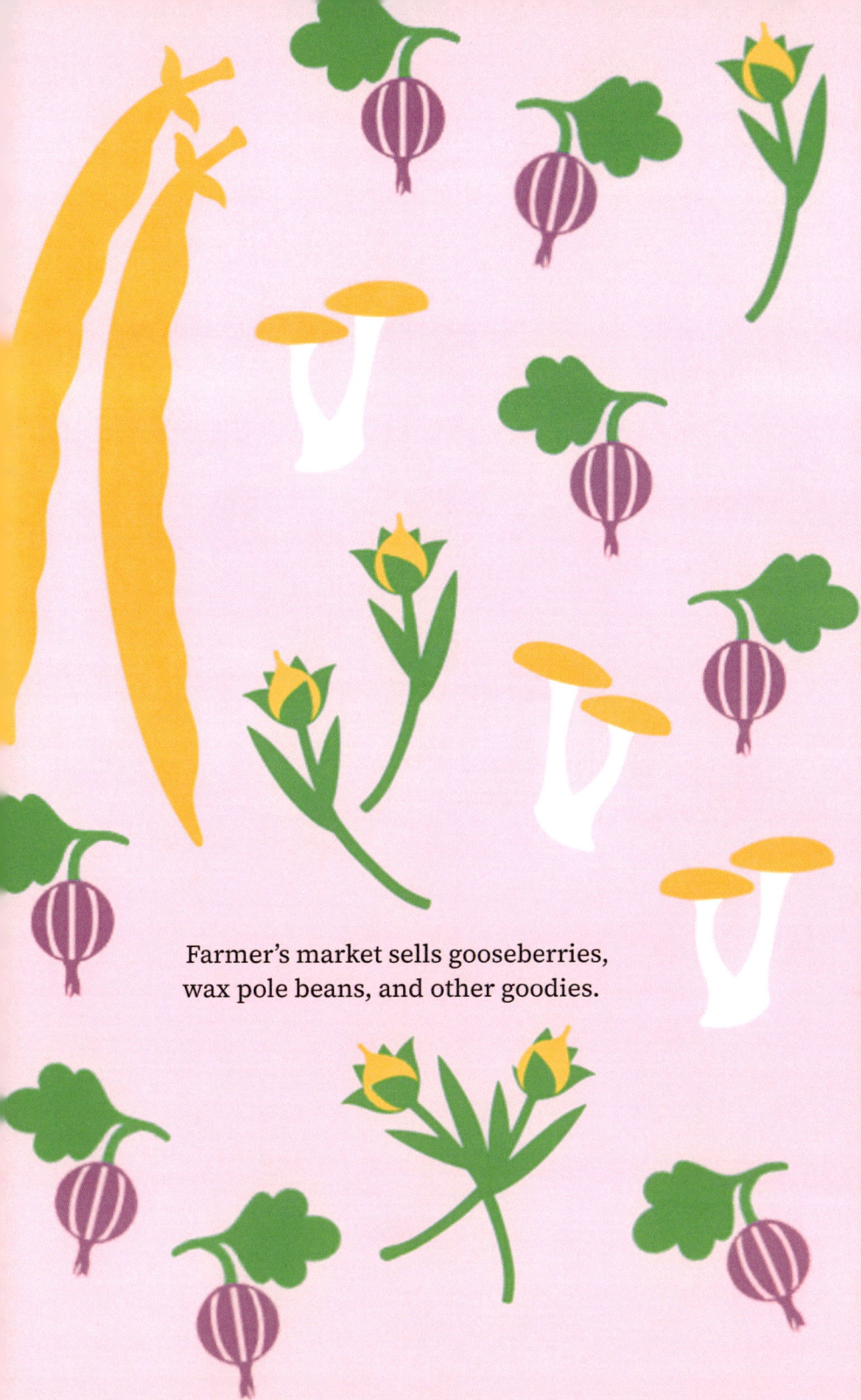

Farmer's market sells gooseberries, wax pole beans, and other goodies.

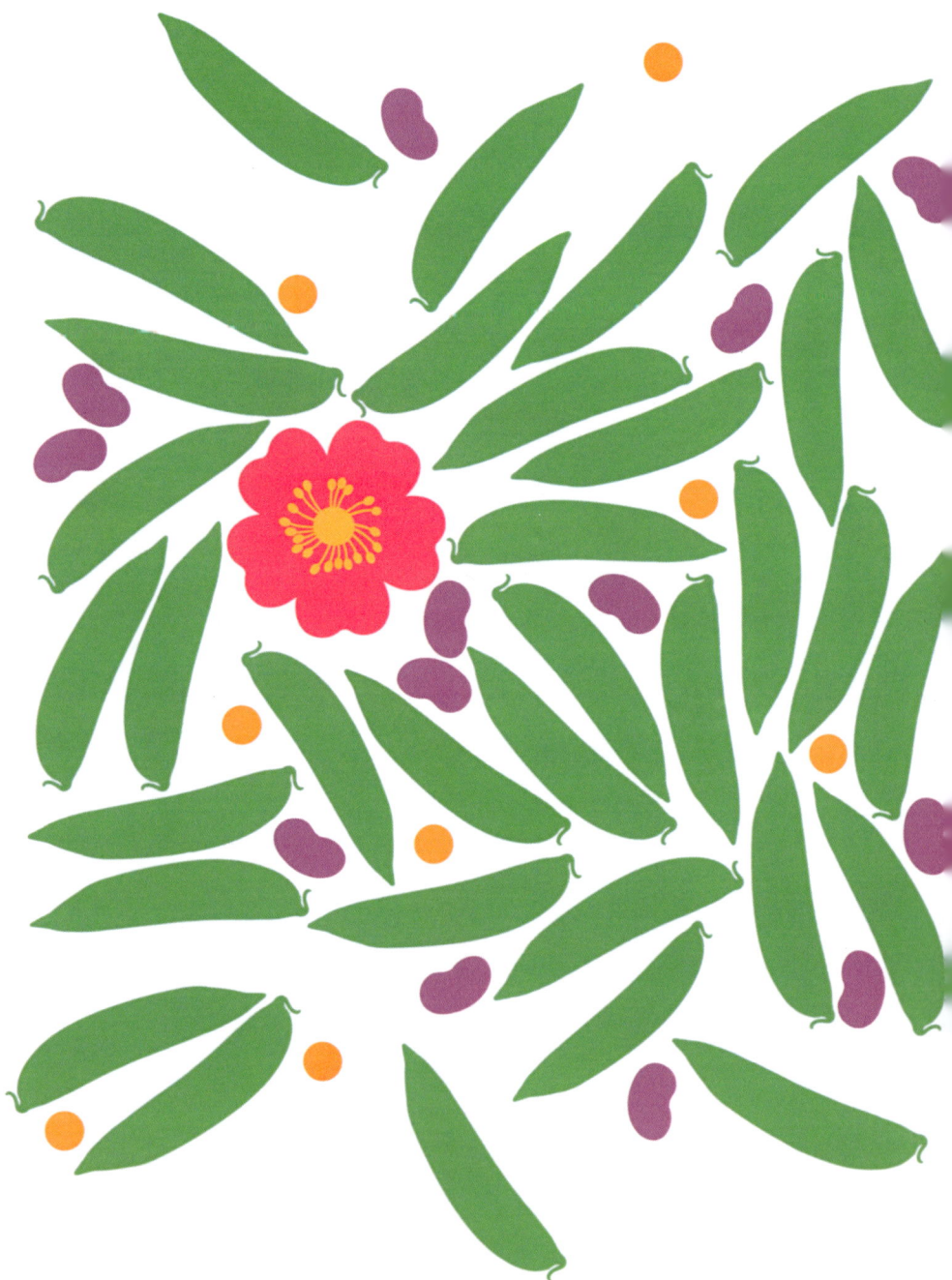

Eat eco-friendly pinto beans,
red lentils, or bright green snow peas.

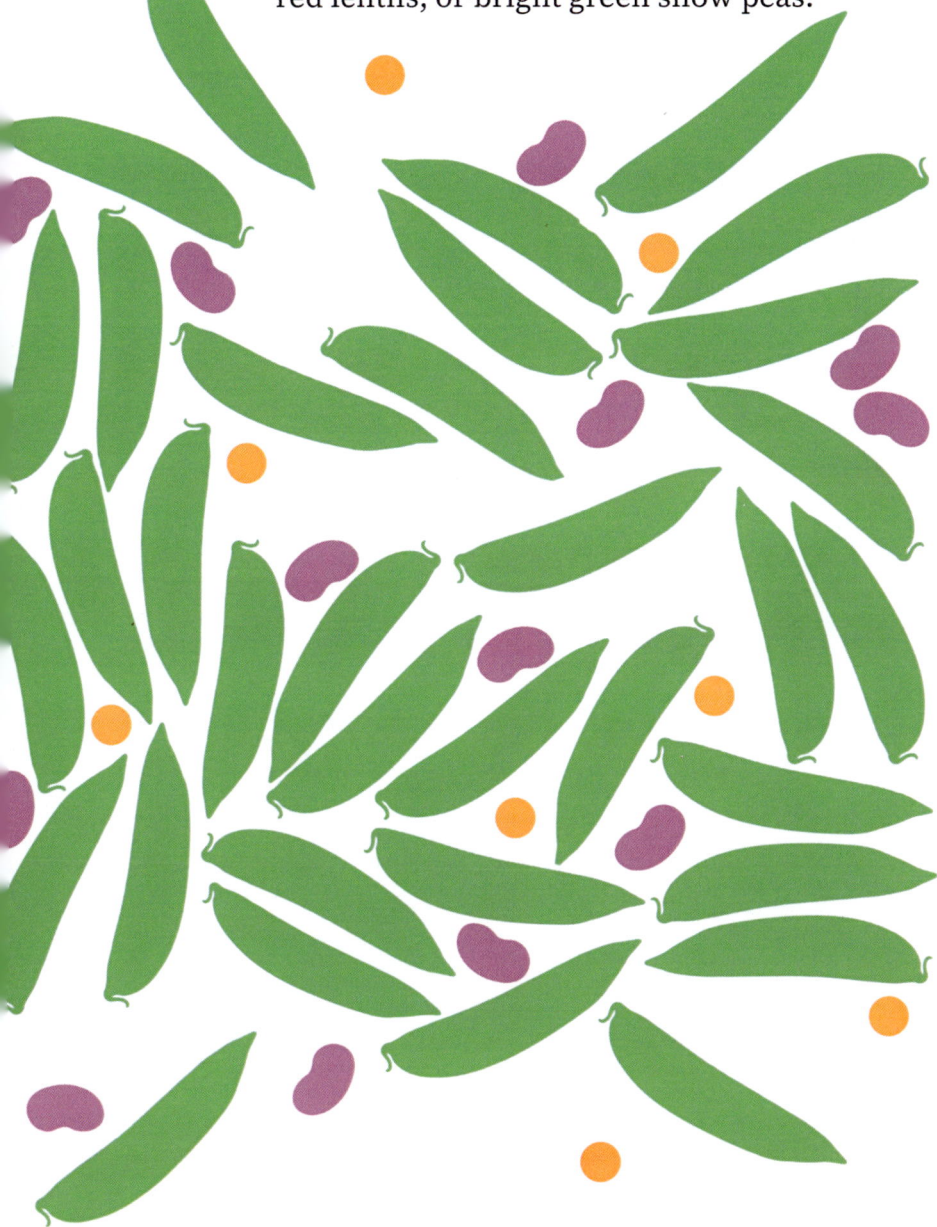

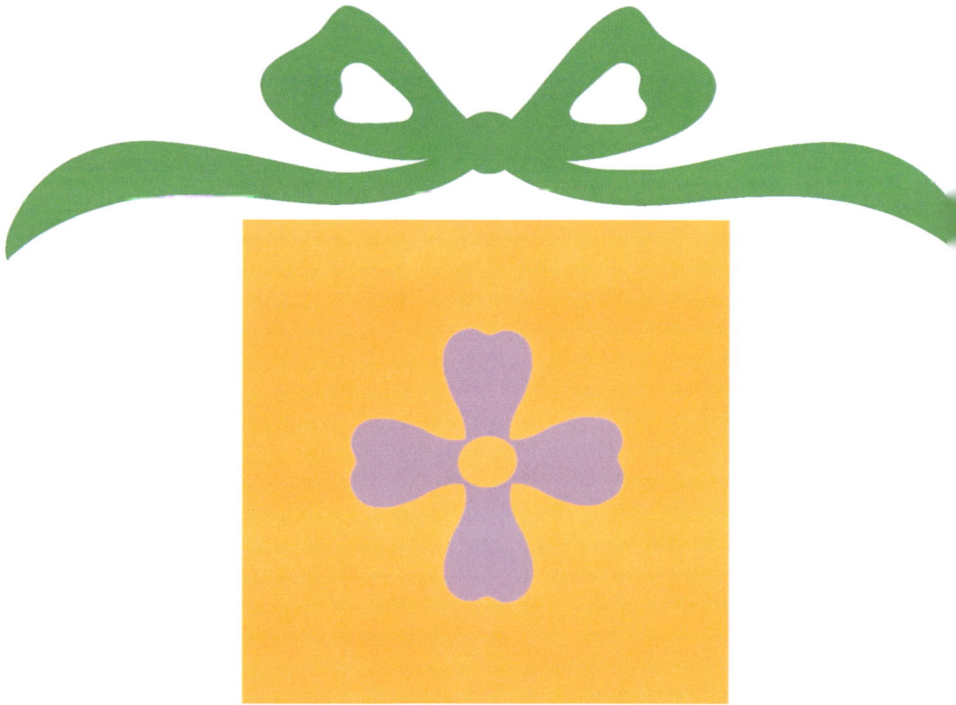

Start an herb box, place where sunny,
grow mint, cilantro, and parsley.

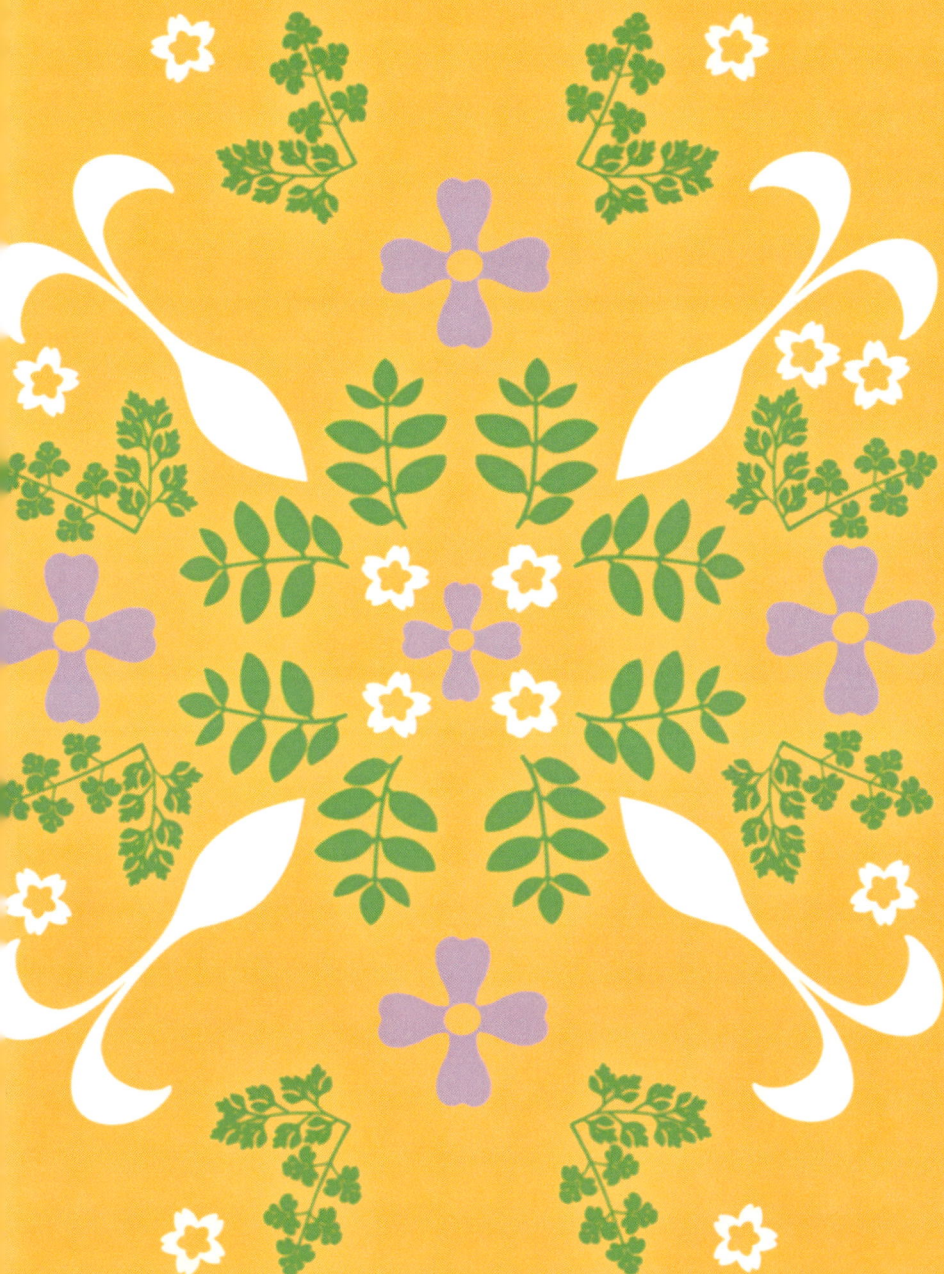

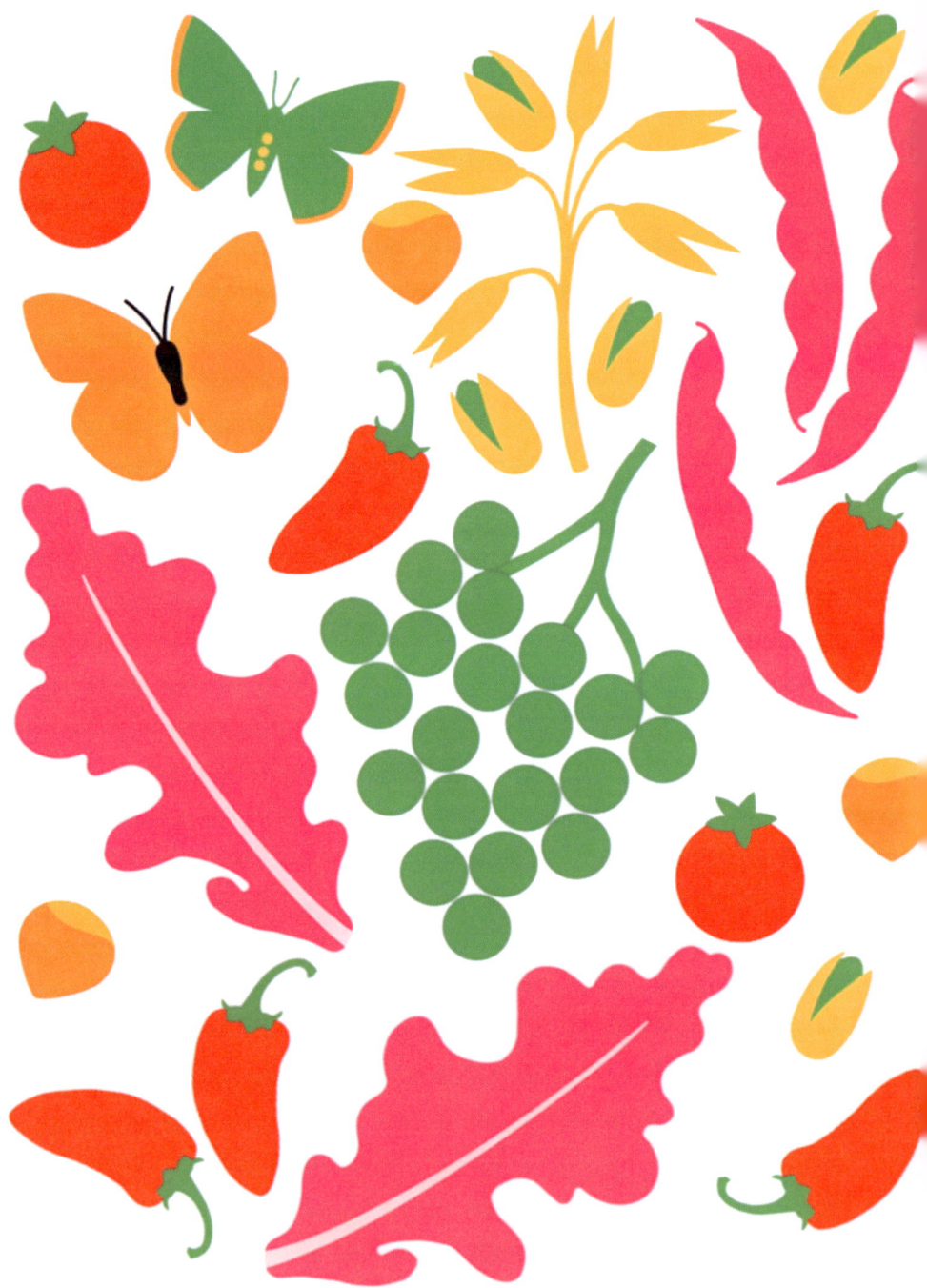

With endless possibilities,
chef's kiss your dish so easily.

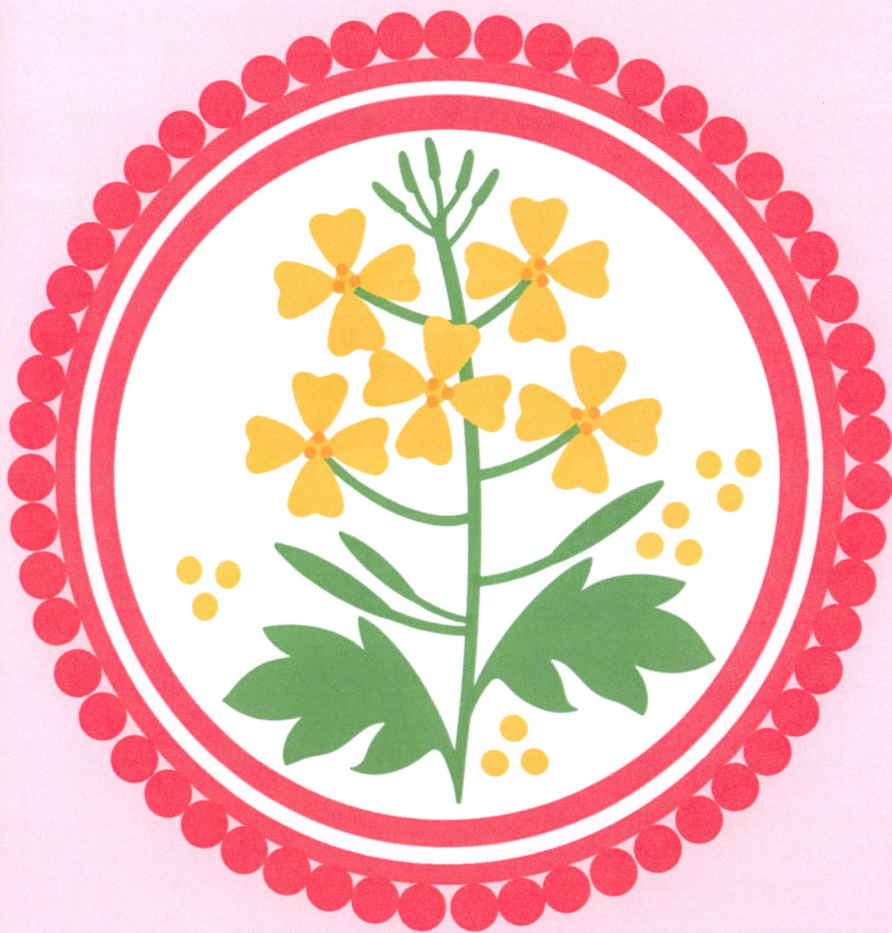

Decorate plates delightfully.
Breakfast becomes a jubilee.
Lunchtime made quite deliciously.

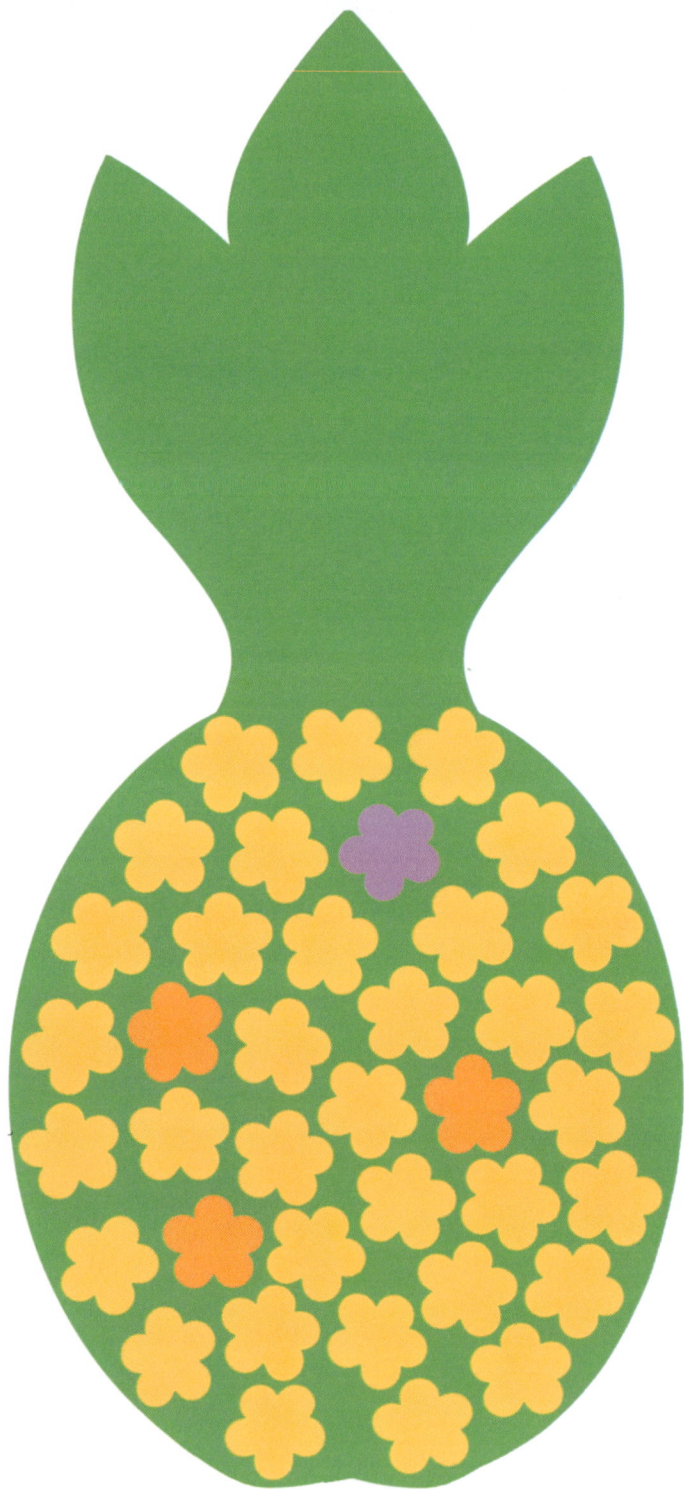

Whether apples or zucchini,
eggplant or pineapple you'll see,
each gift from God as heavenly.

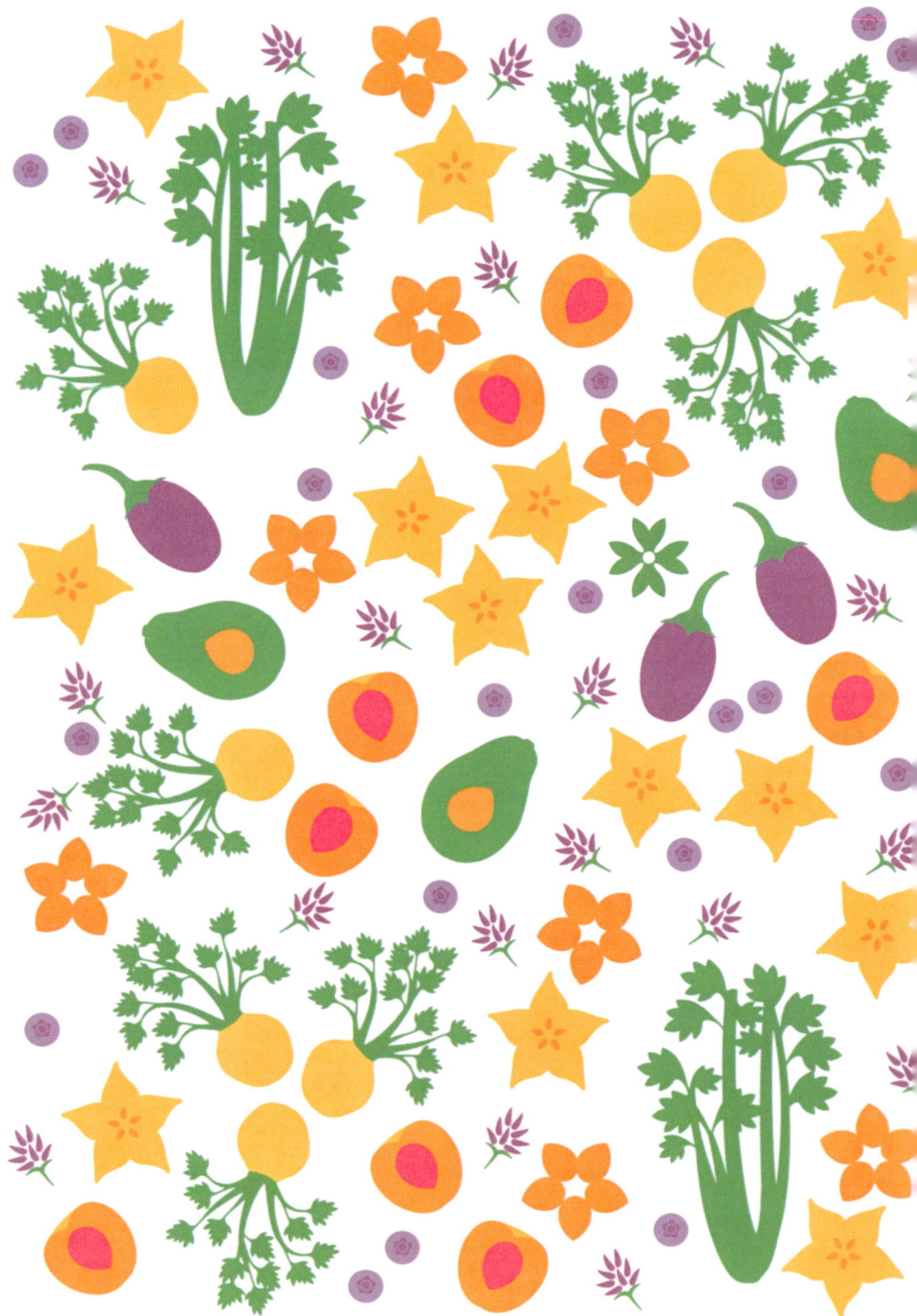

Gardens produce fine symphonies:
each note is from God, honestly.

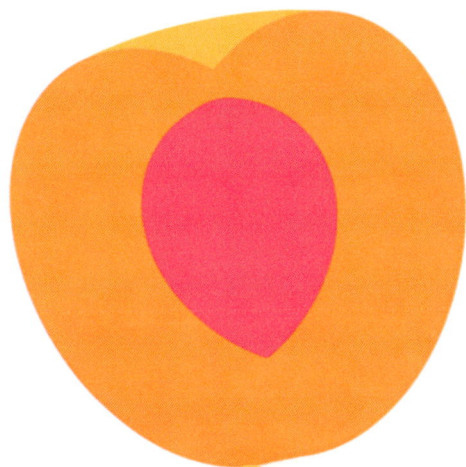

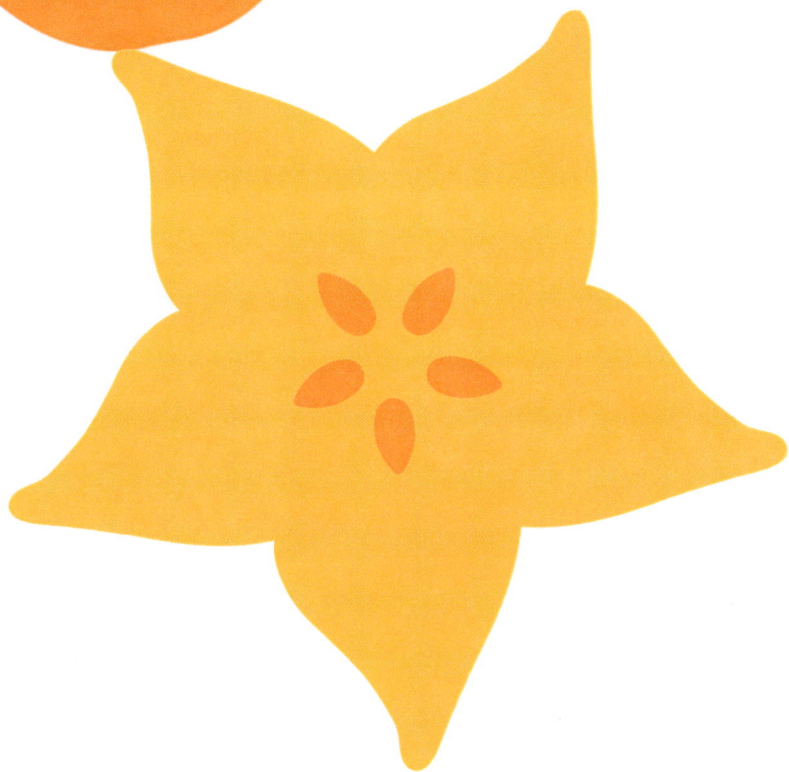

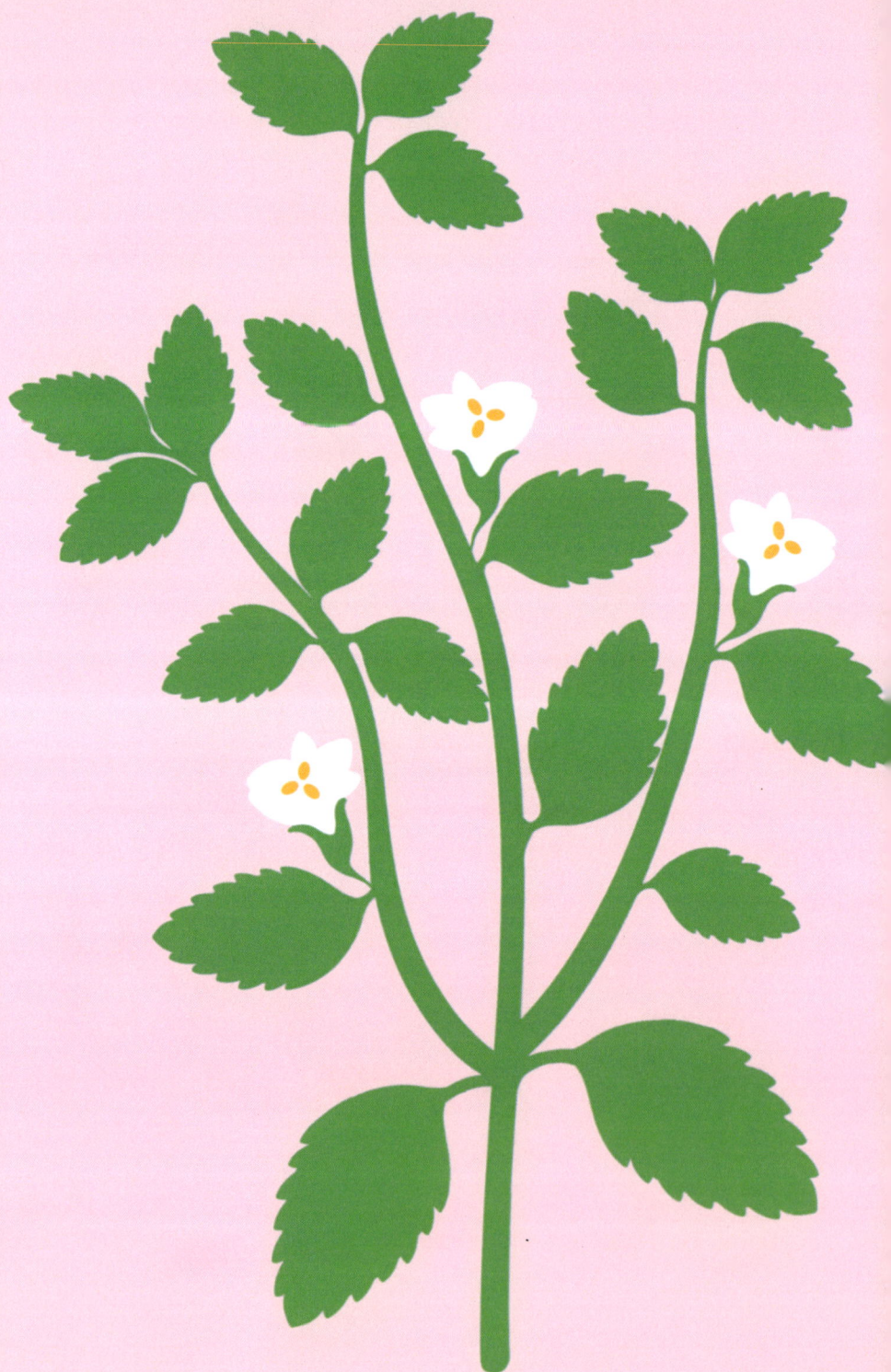

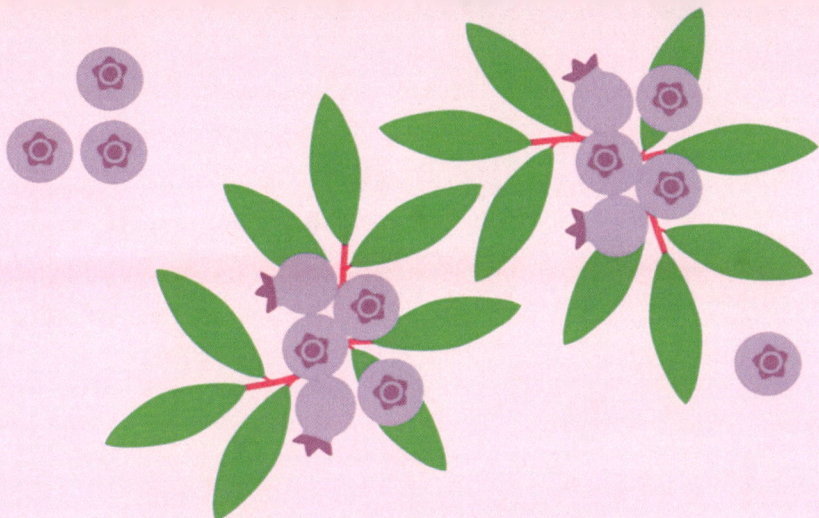

Angels follow fine recipes.
Start with grace, end with remedies.
Food as medicine stops disease.

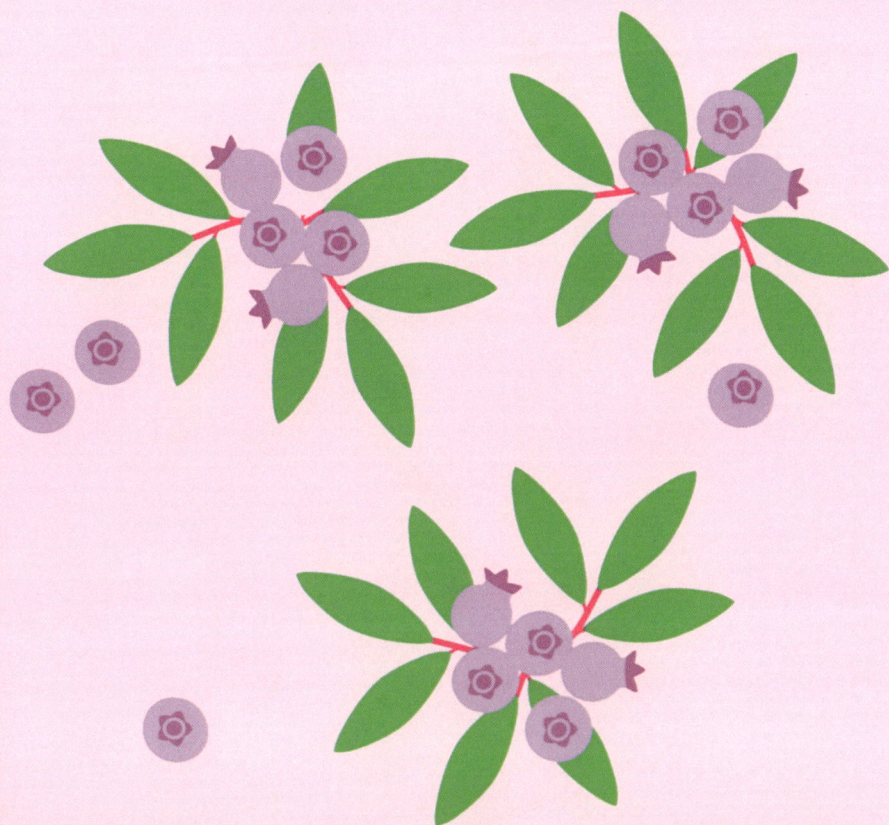

A superfood:
goji berries.

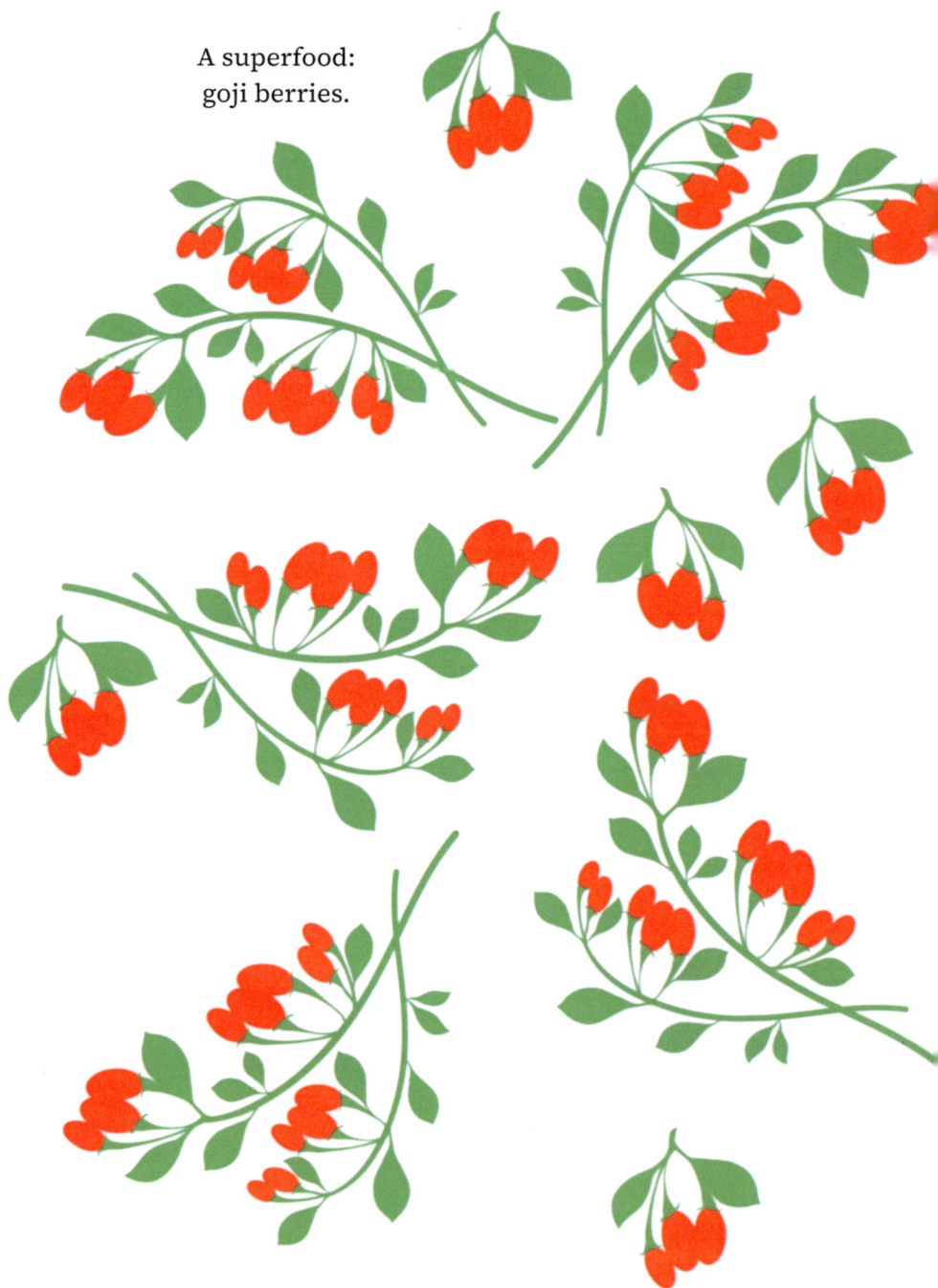

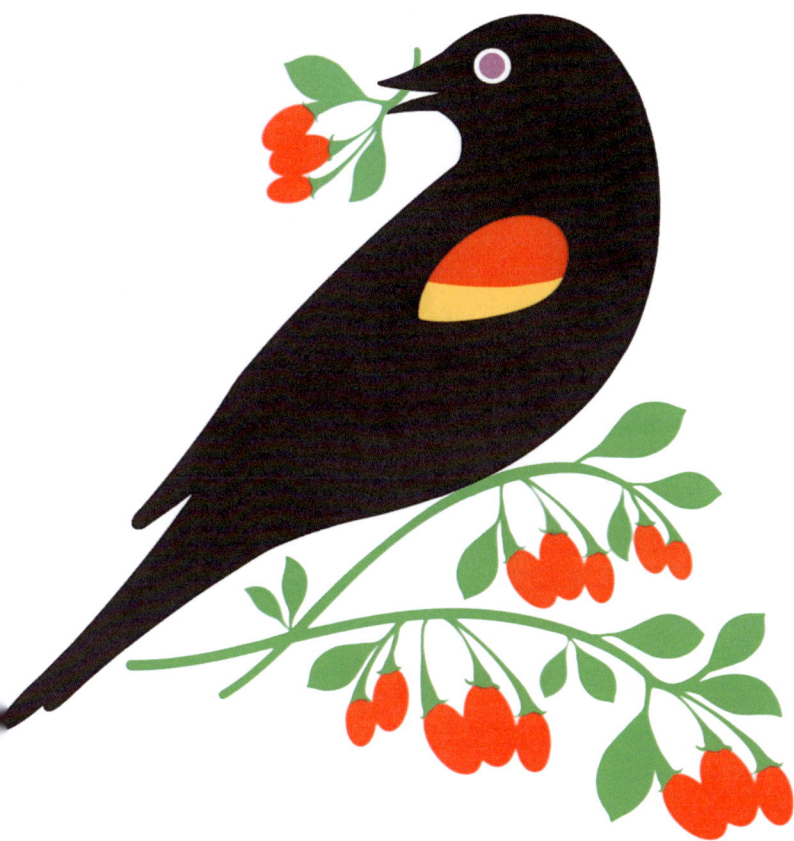

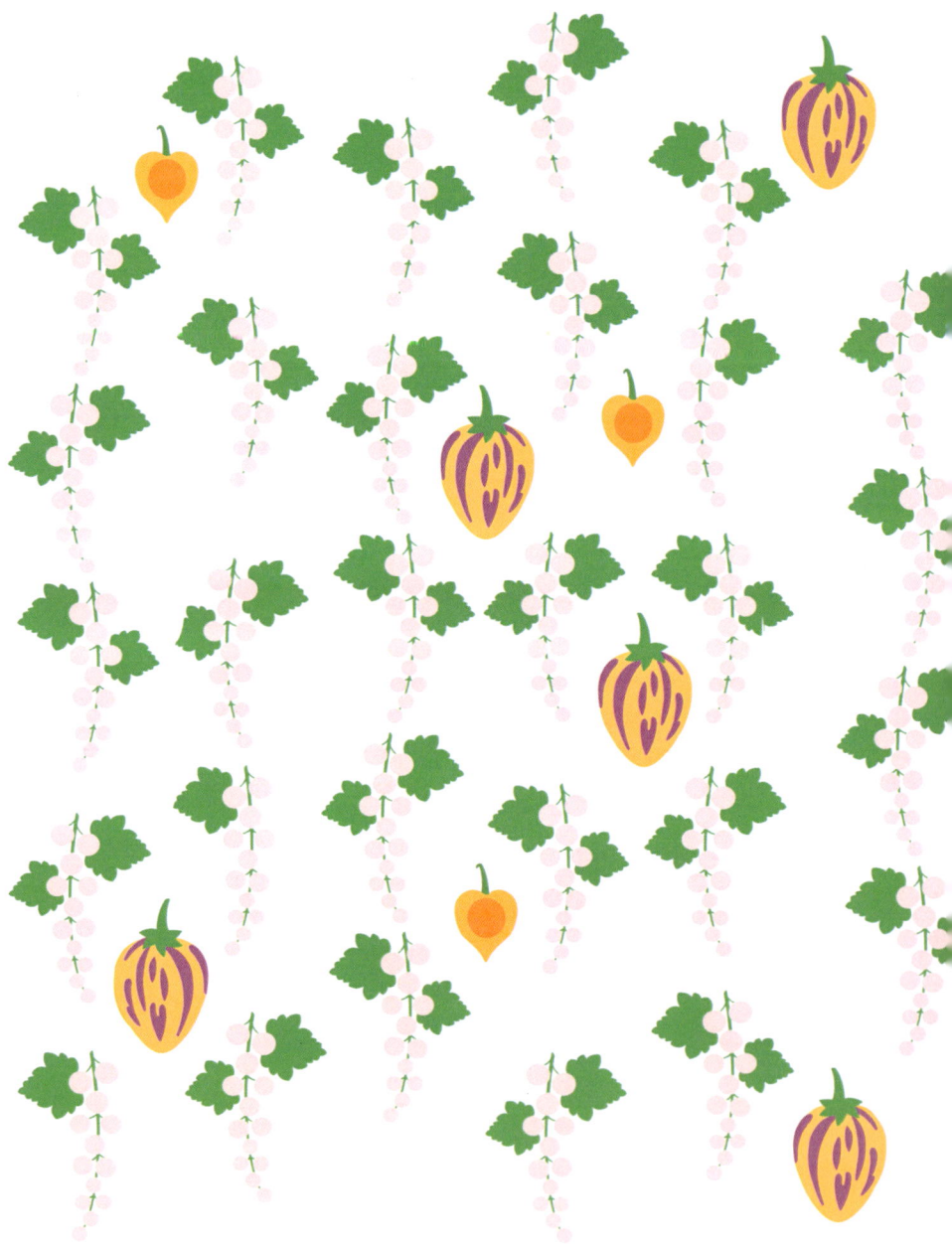

There is an amazing medley,
fun yet nourishing, certainly.

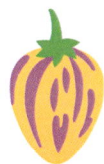

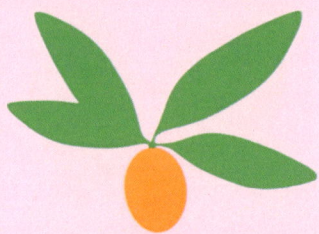

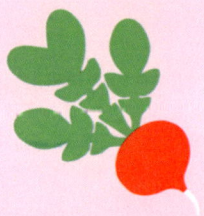

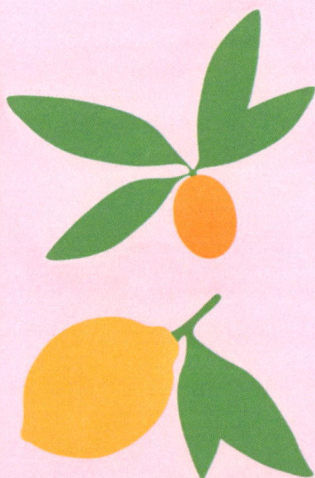

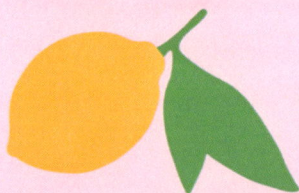

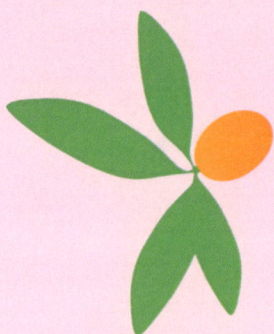

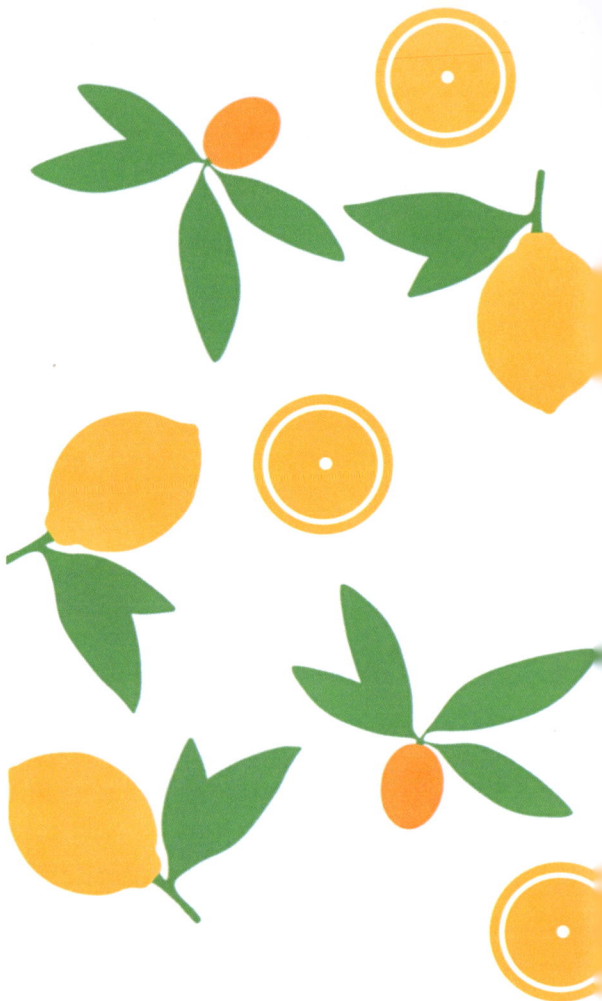

Little kumquats taste so tangy.
Crisp radishes are quite spicy.
Yellow lemons stay so zesty.

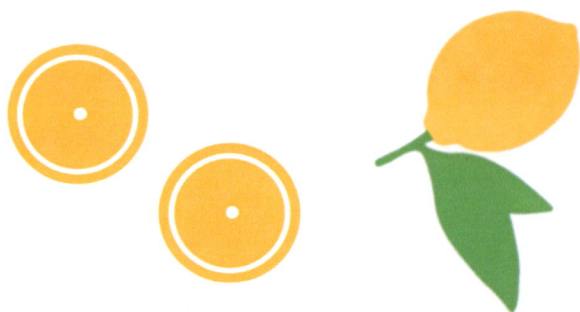

Spinach awards vitality.
Get guavas for immunity.
Try cabbage for longevity.

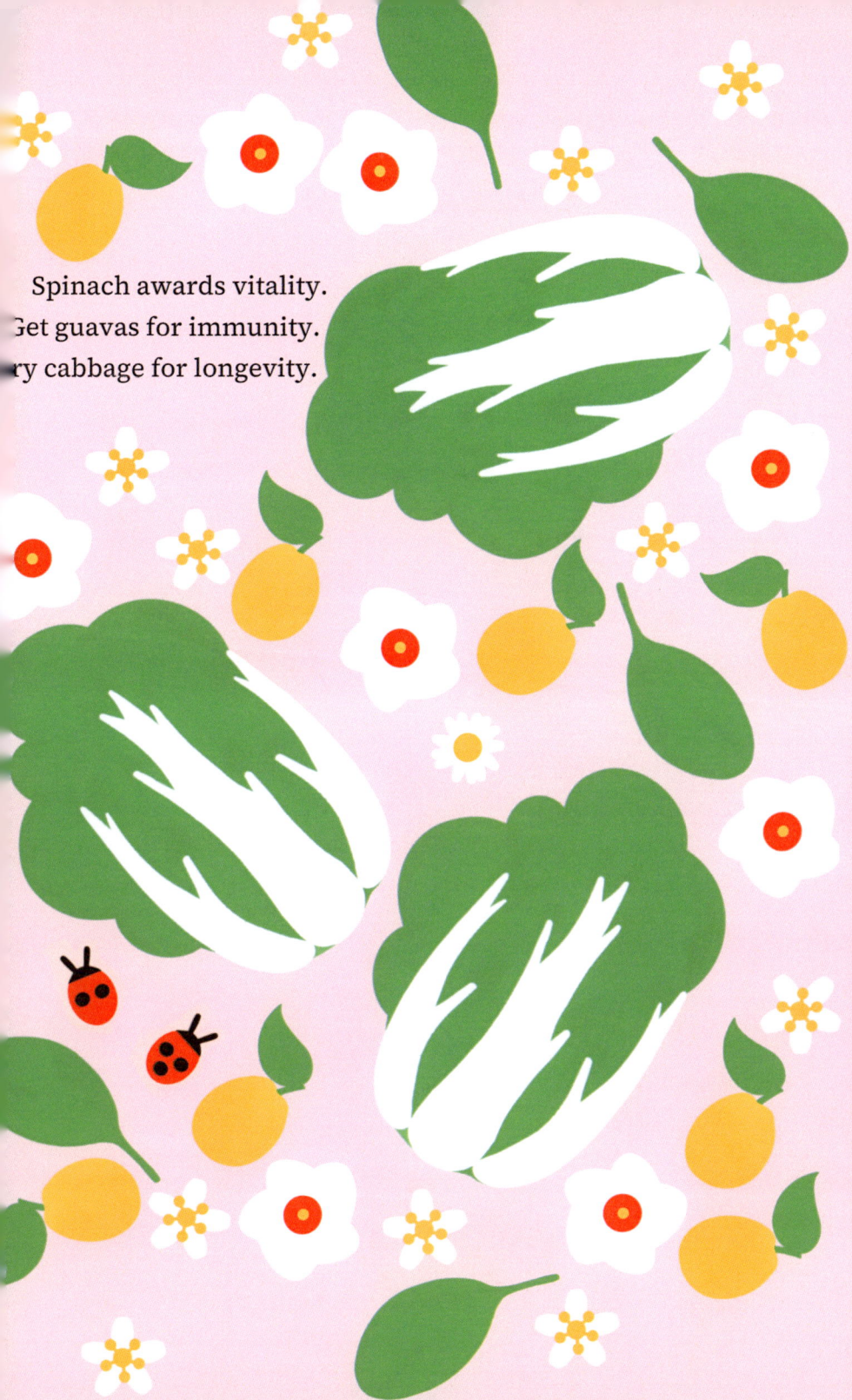

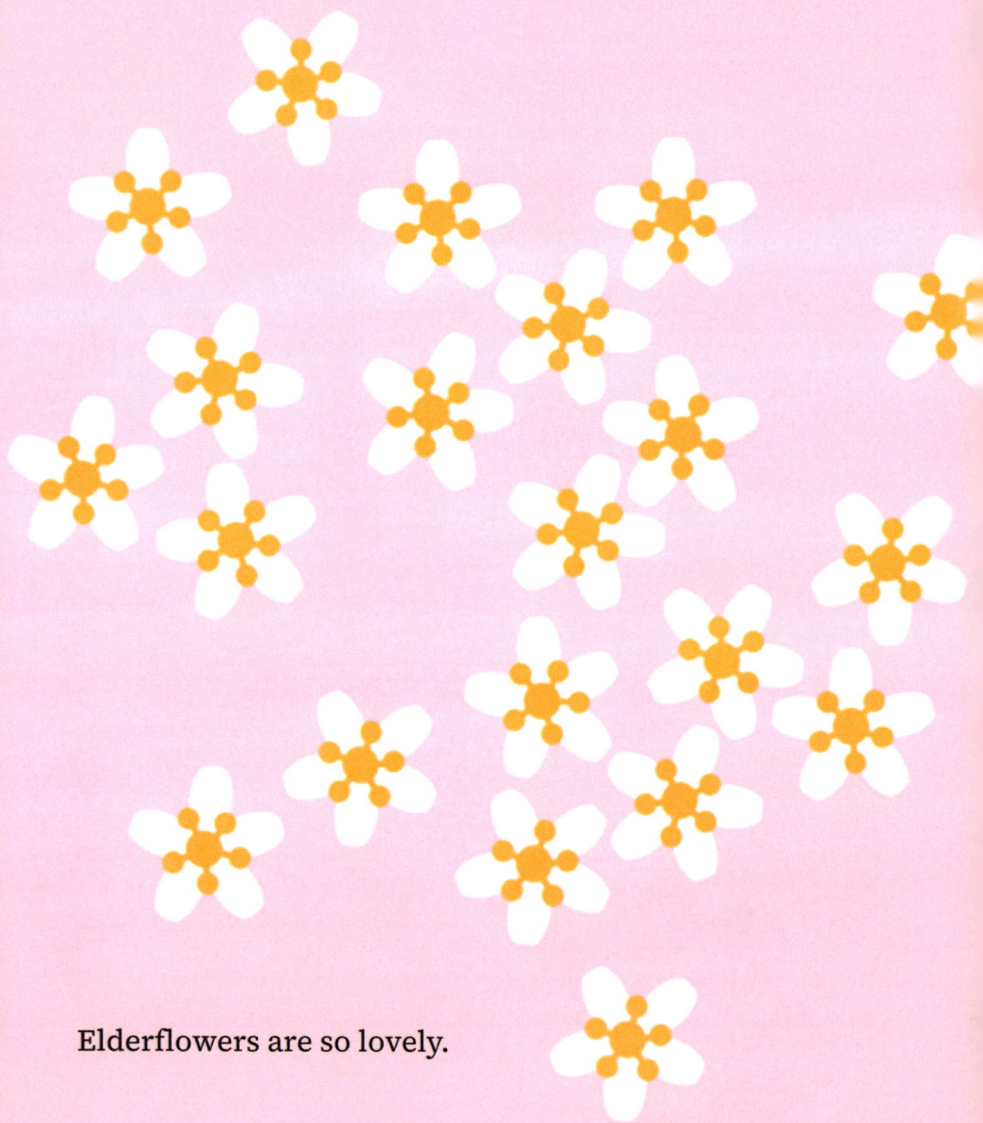

Elderflowers are so lovely.

Citrus wheels positivity.

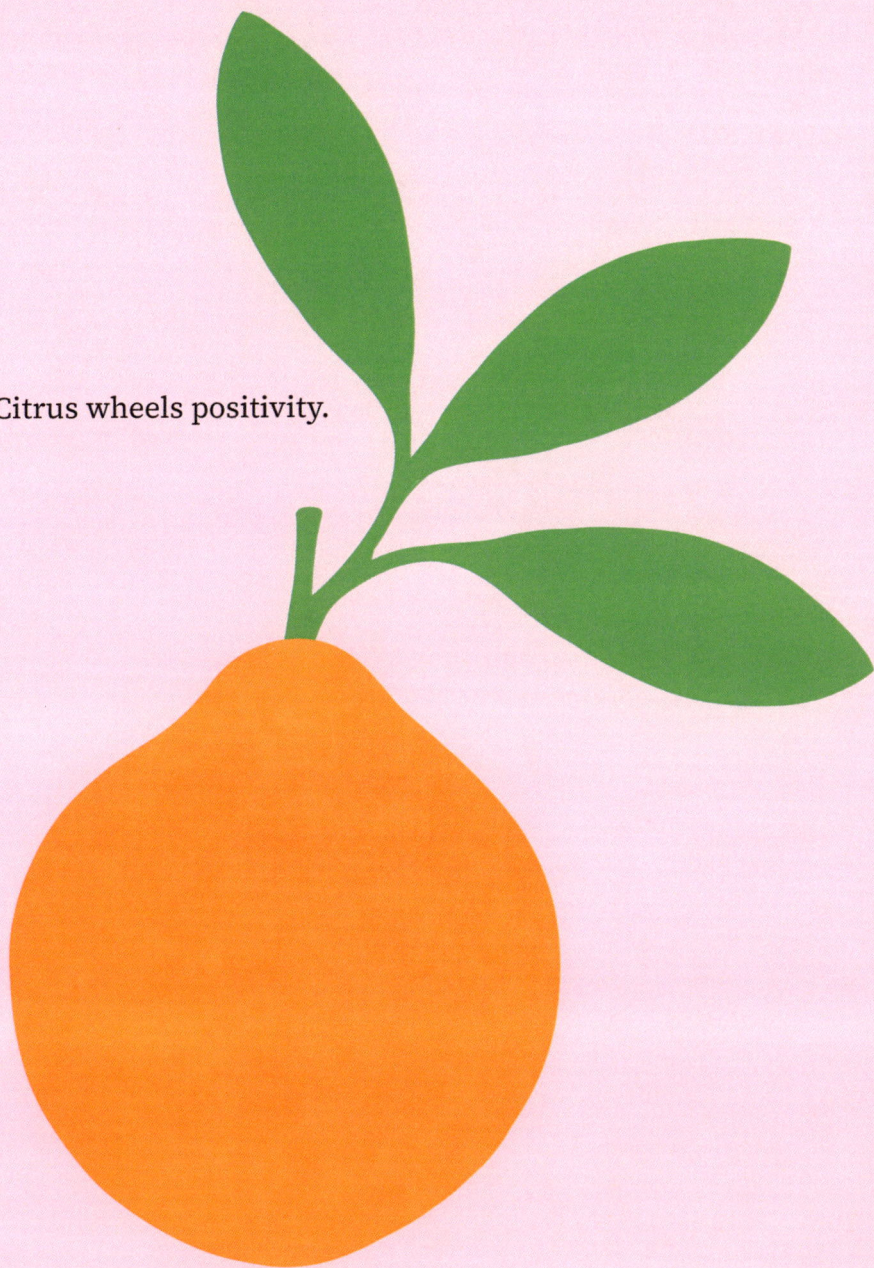

Jicama, more than just crunchy.
It's low in fat and calorie.

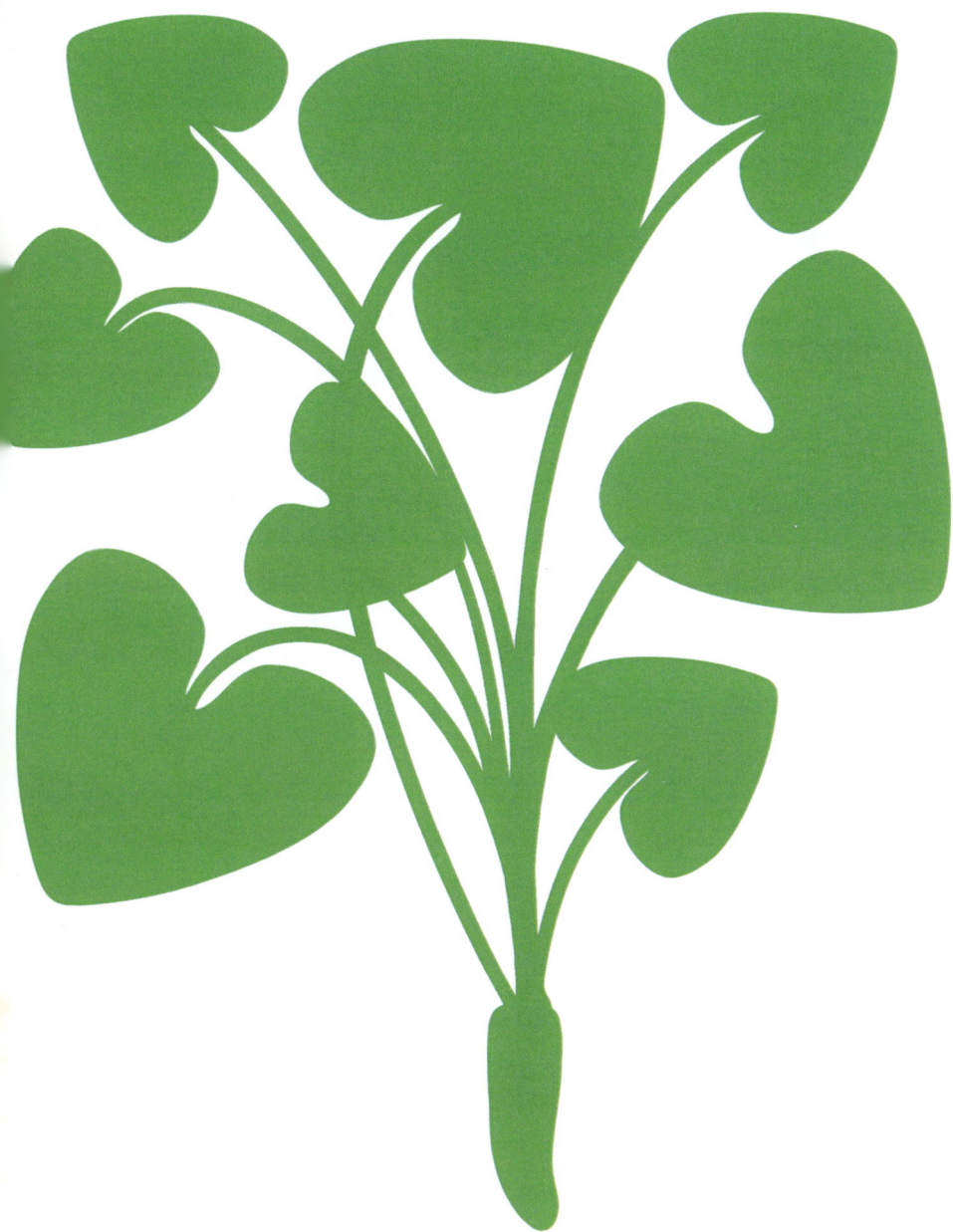

Surprisingly hot: wasabi.

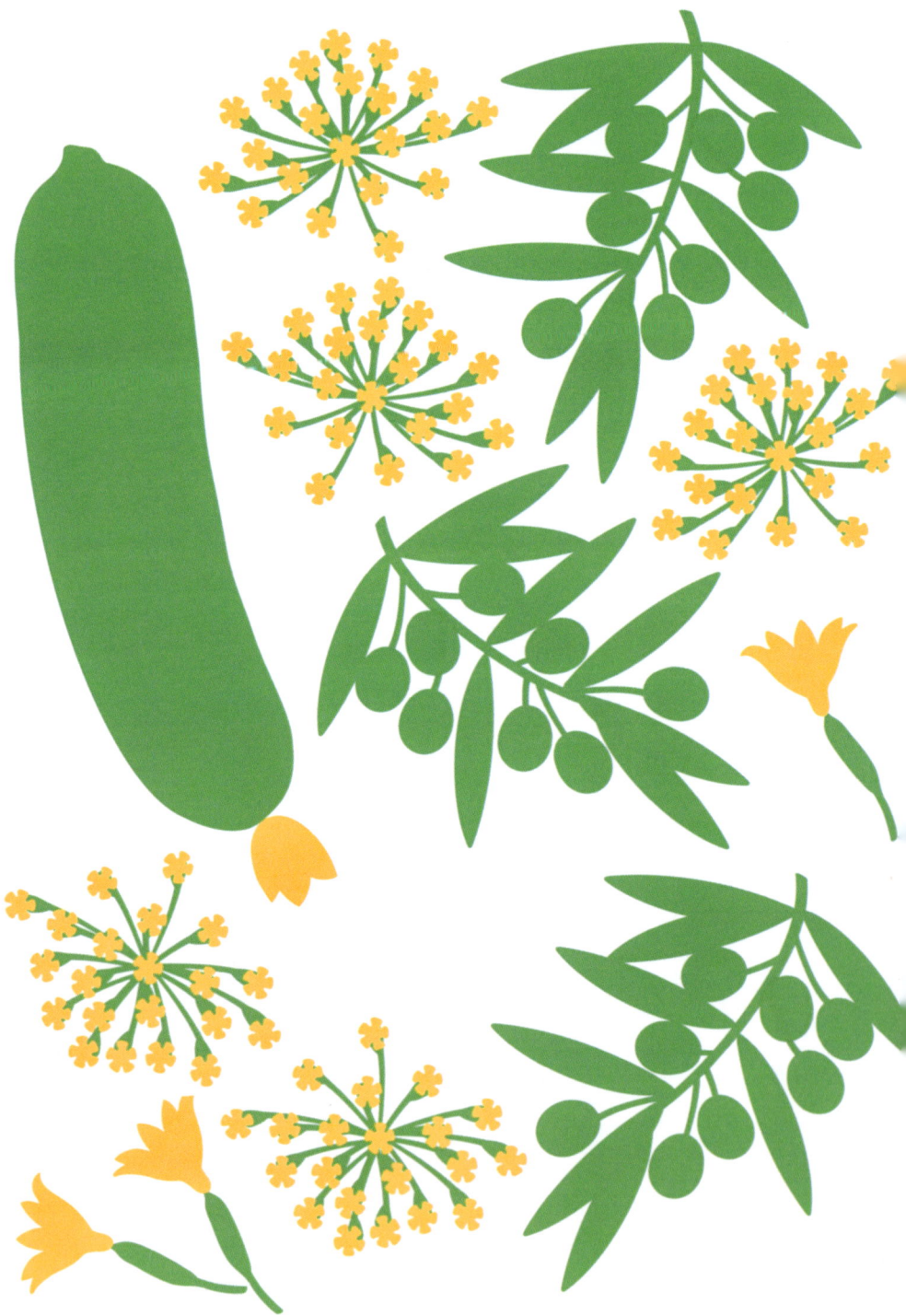

od already made crops healthy.
nswers are found in history.
Make prosperity your story.

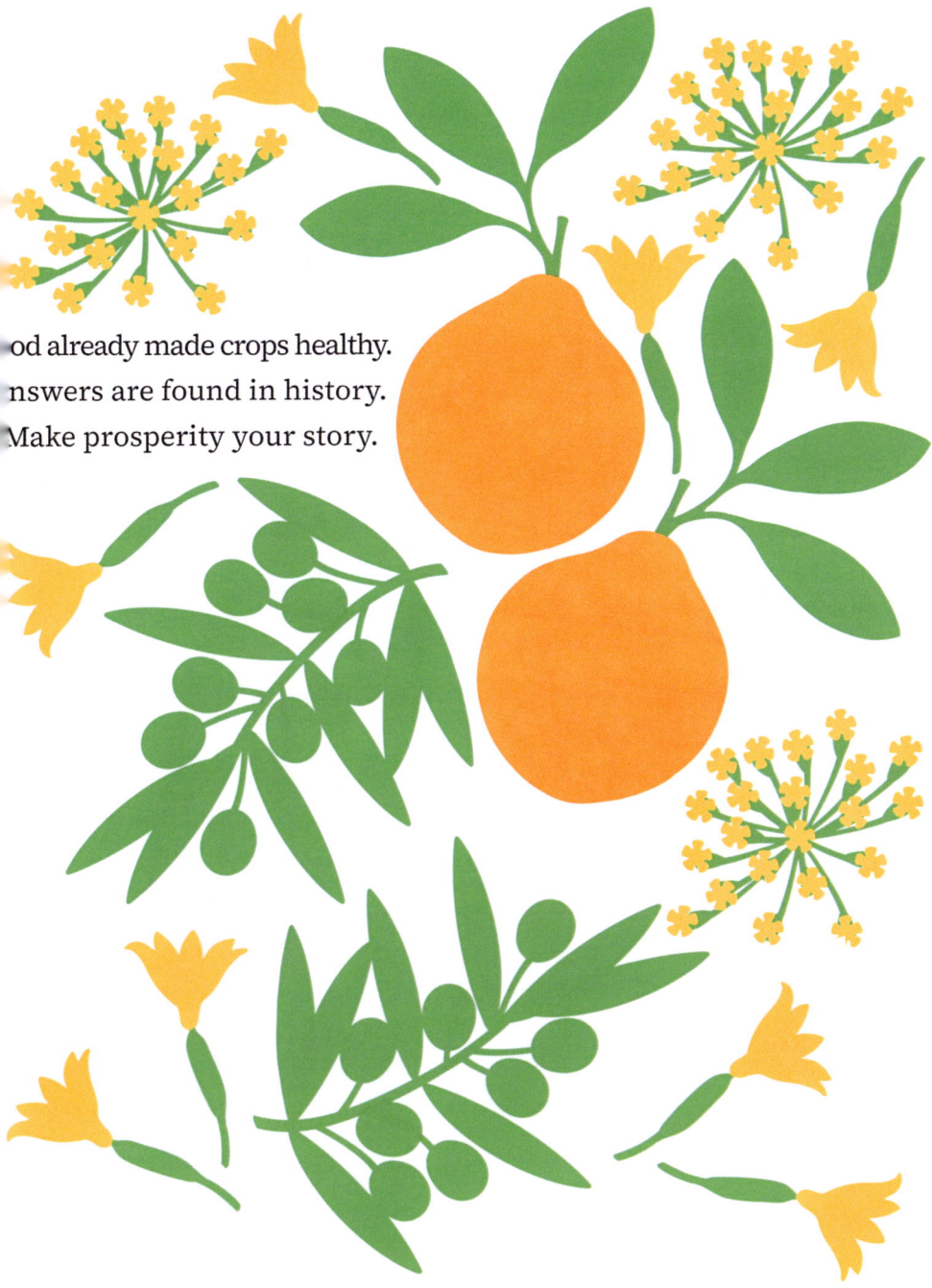

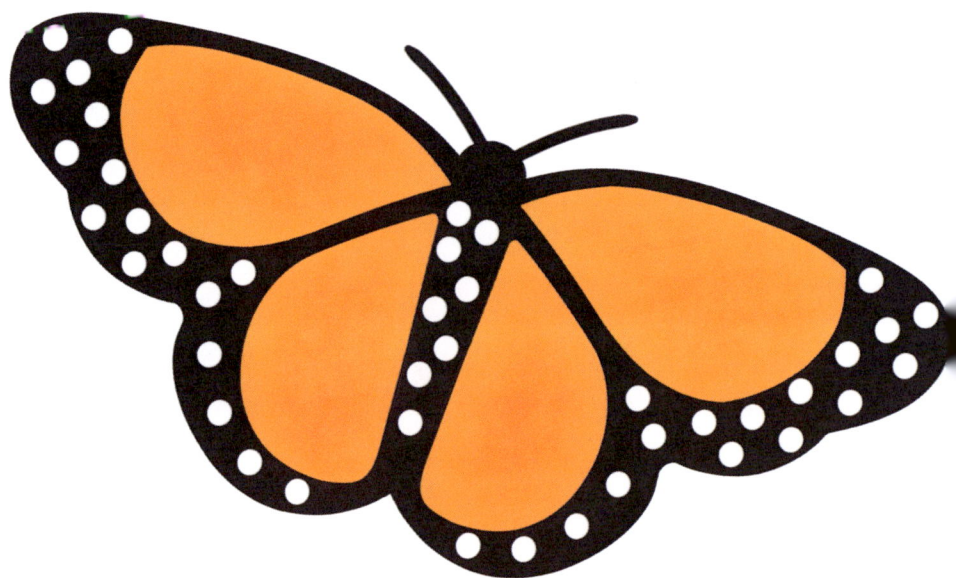

God's creatures, worthy of glory.

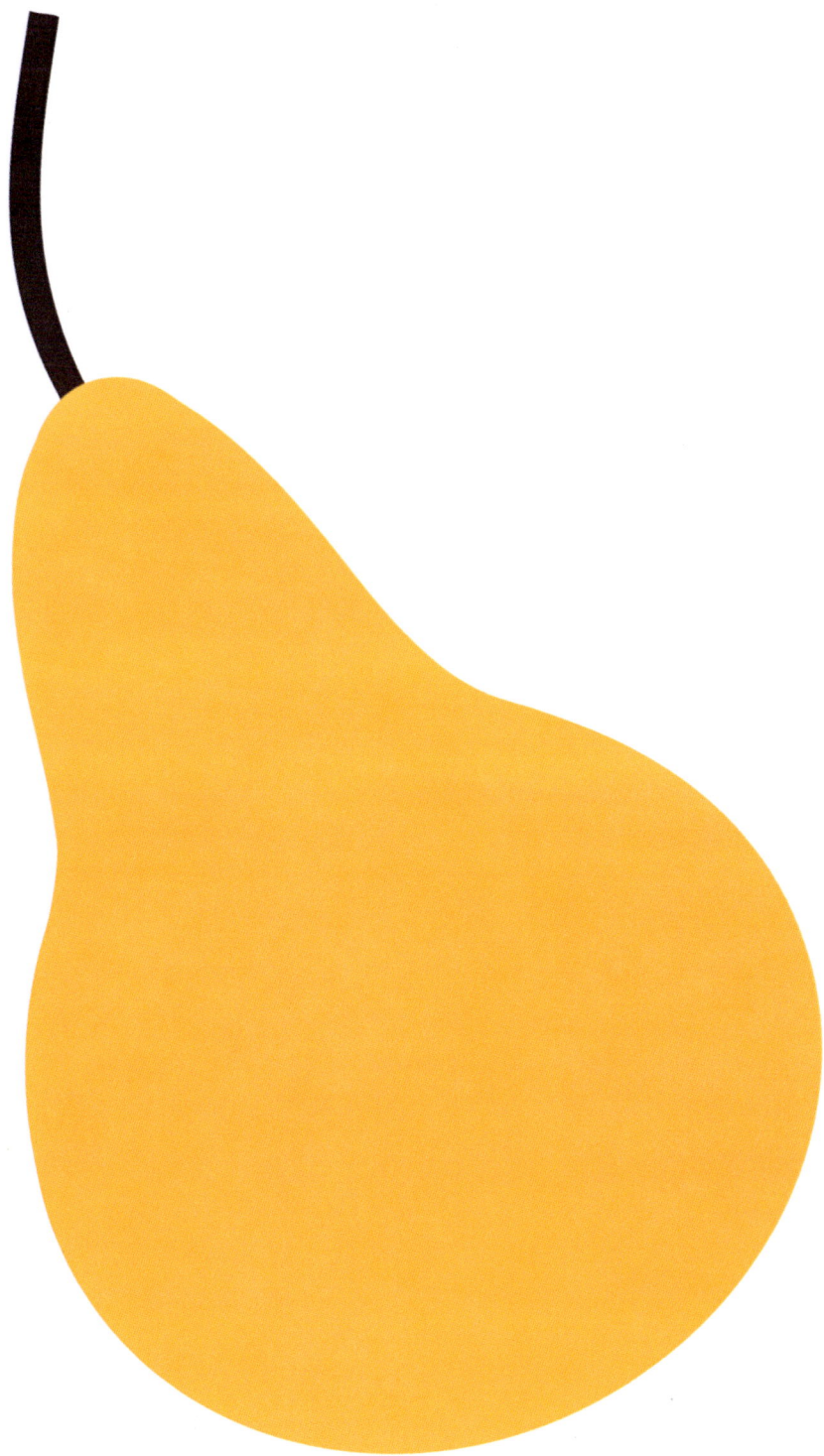

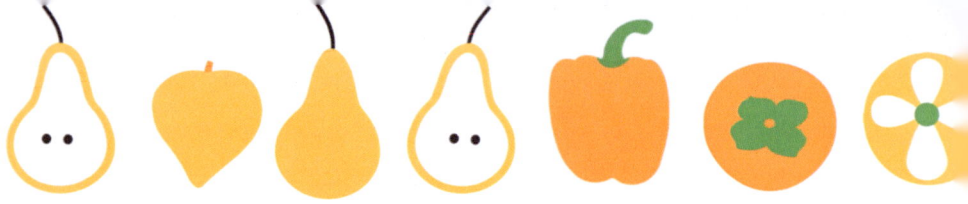

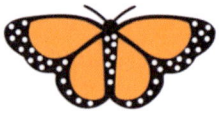

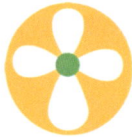

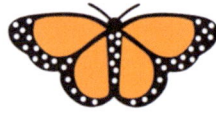

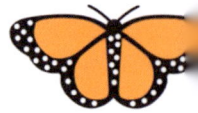

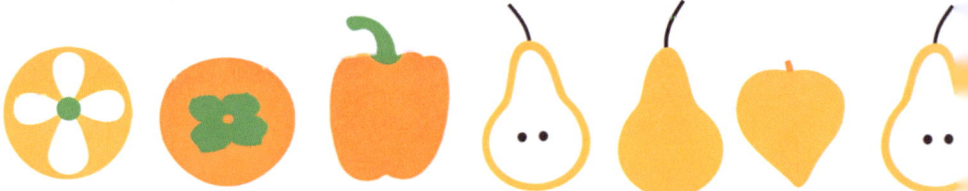

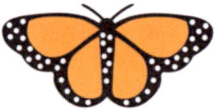

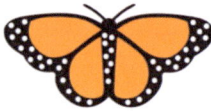

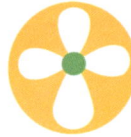

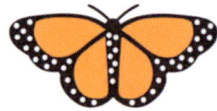

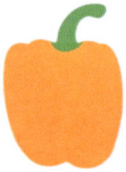

In a world where all grows wholly,
crops will bloom so bright and fully,
flavored only naturally,
not ever artificially.

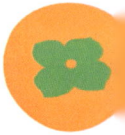

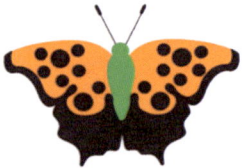

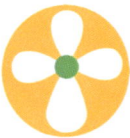

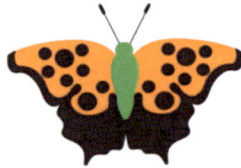

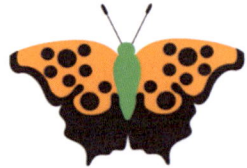

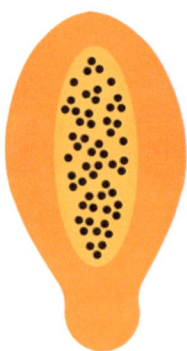

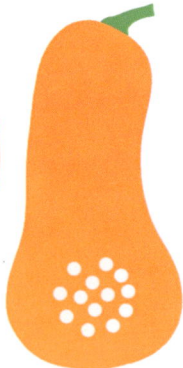

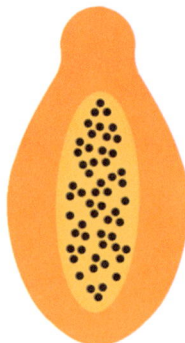

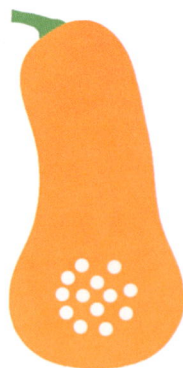

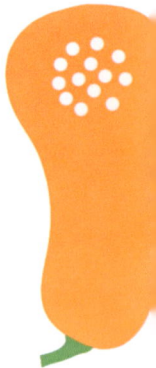

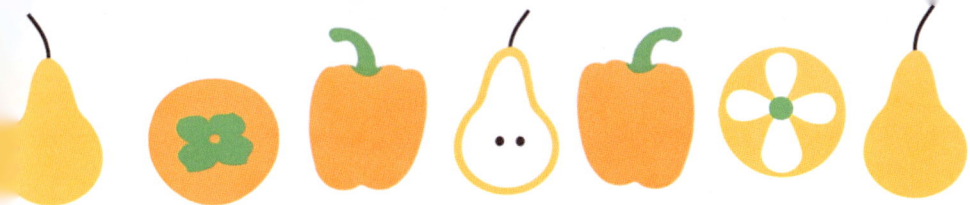

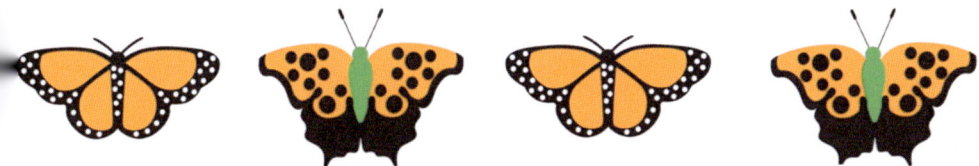

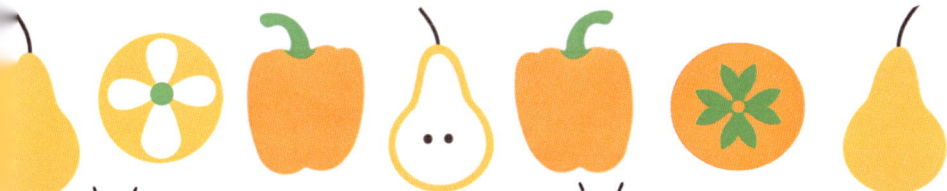

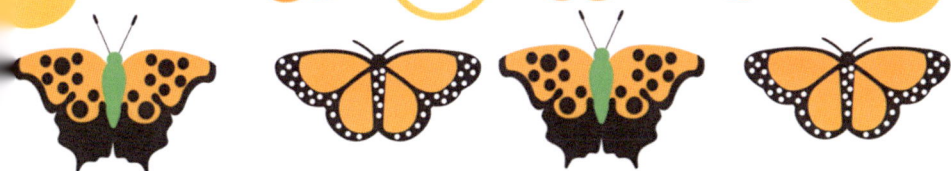

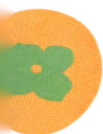

We'll appreciate finally,
fruits and vegetables aplenty,
for myself and everybody.

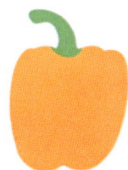

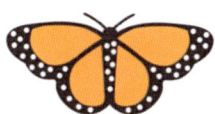

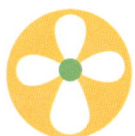

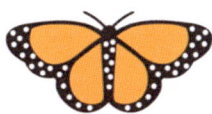

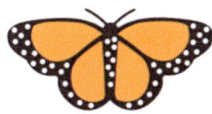

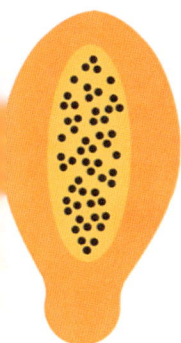

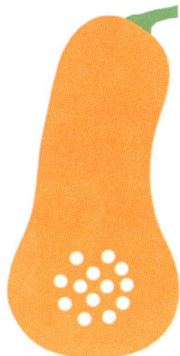

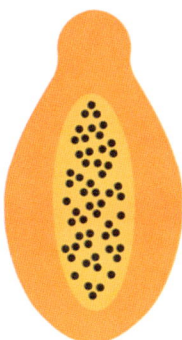

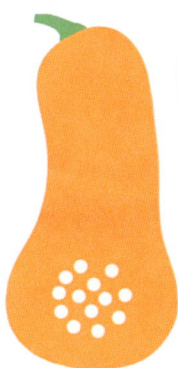

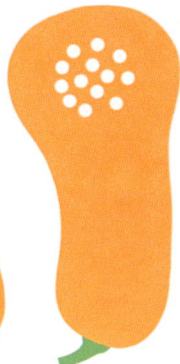

Pears, prickly
and elderberries.

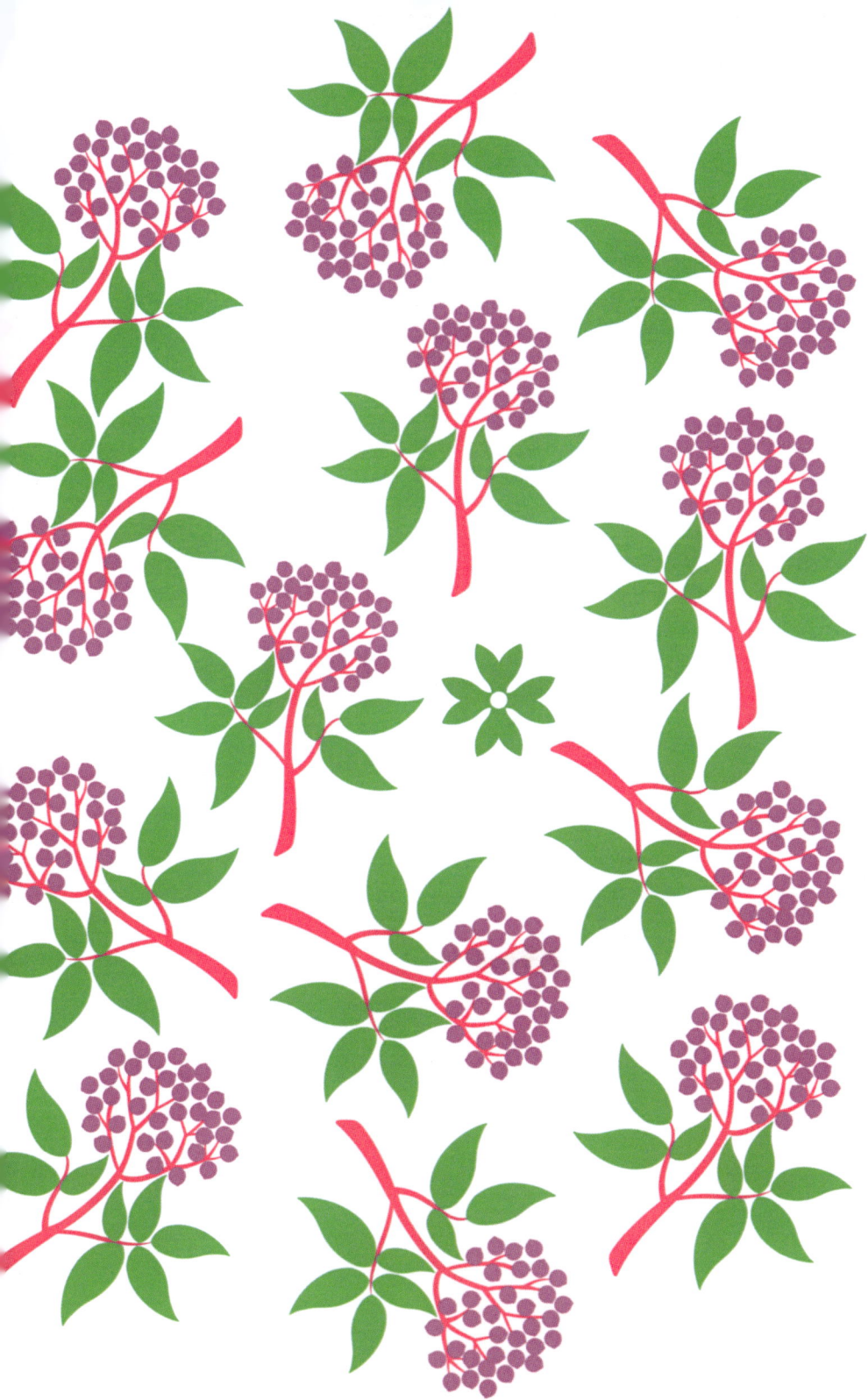

Food is precious, act faithfully.

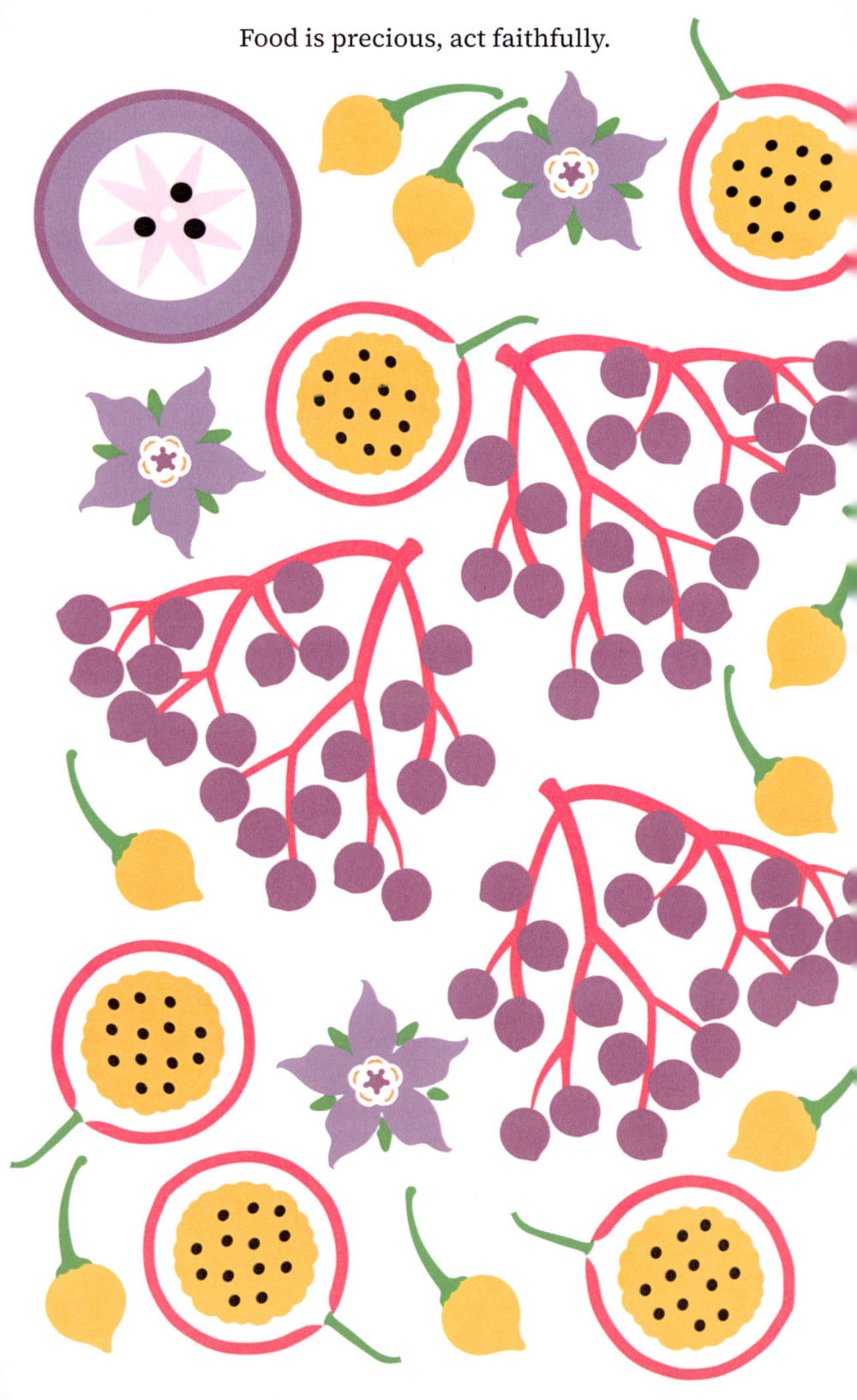

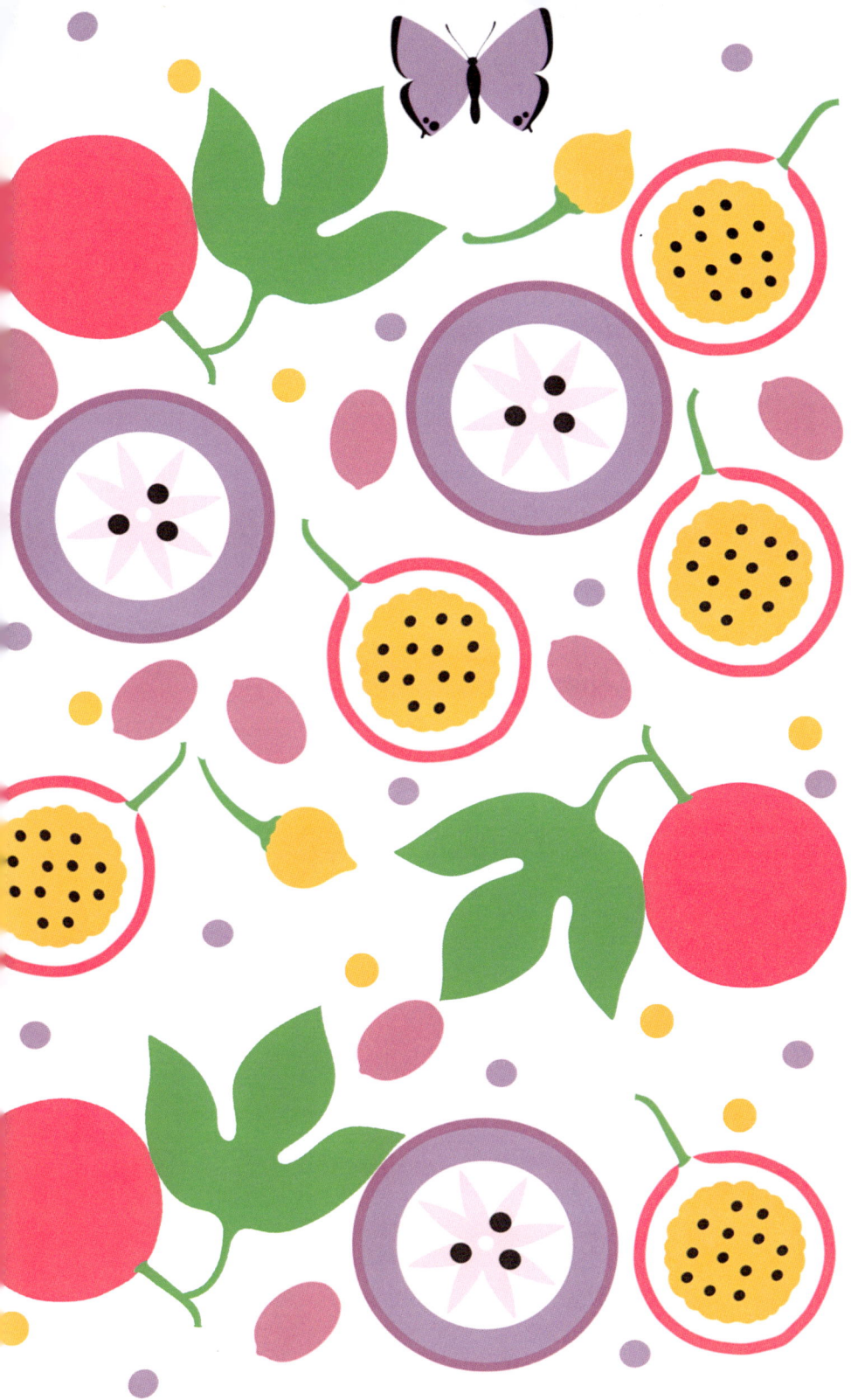

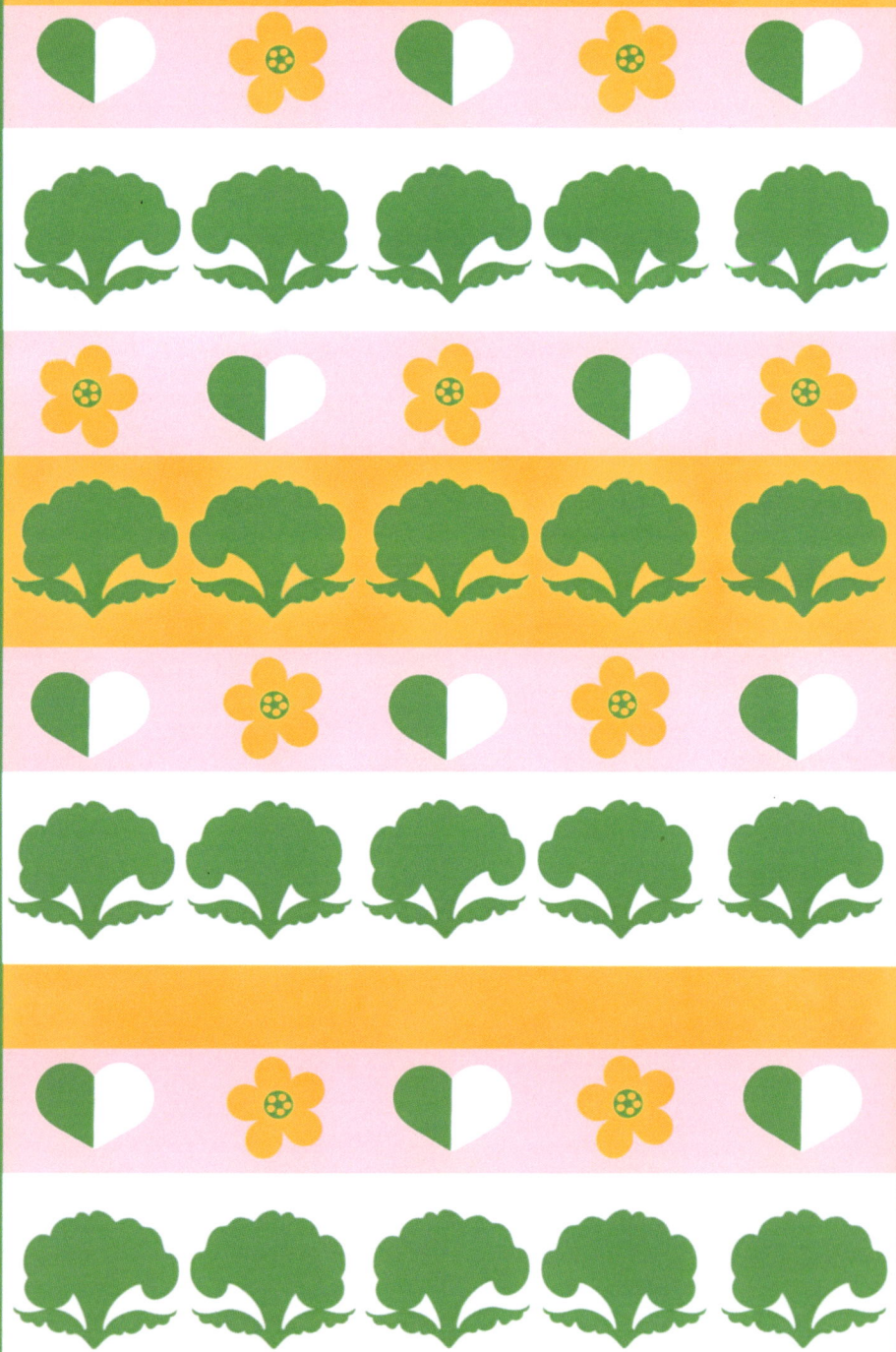

We can say thanks with poetry,
in many words or just simply:
Dear Lord, "Please bless my broccoli,"
with love and full sincerity.

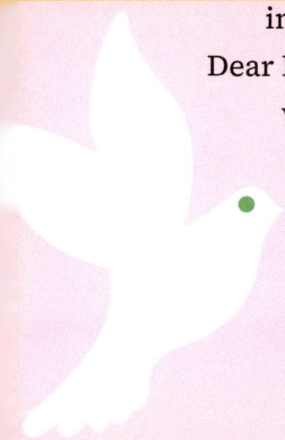

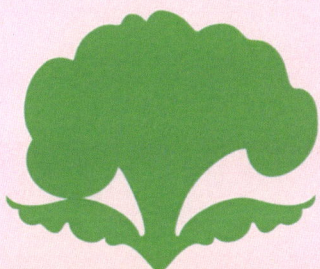

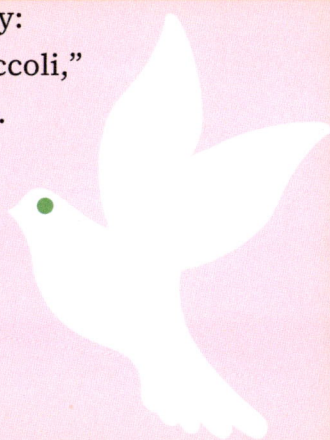

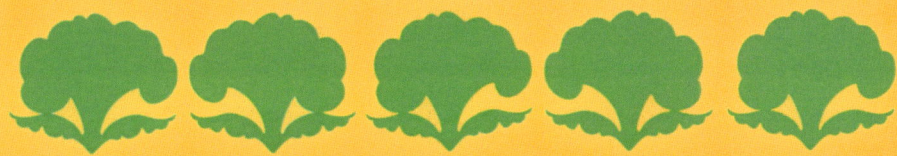

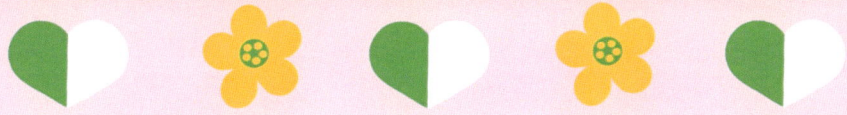

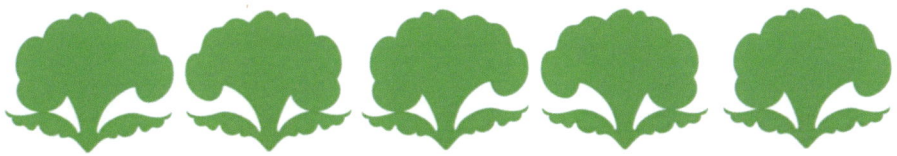

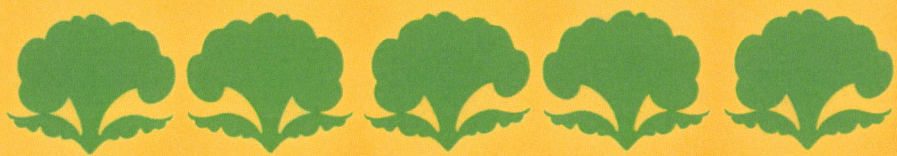

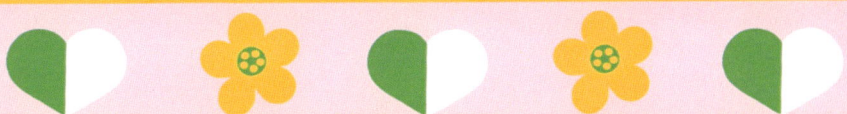

Bonus page here, most thoughtfully.
Thank you, God, for all you give me.
I'll share with joy and harmony.
For those who love poems and scenes,
enjoy charming rose-like lychees.

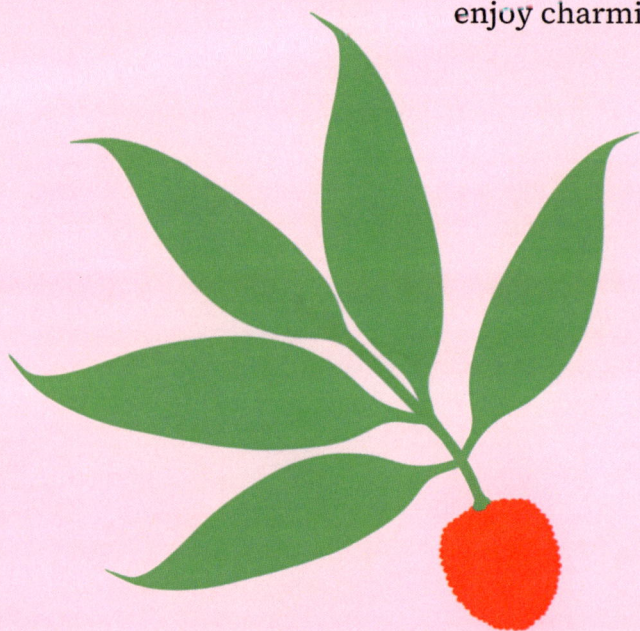

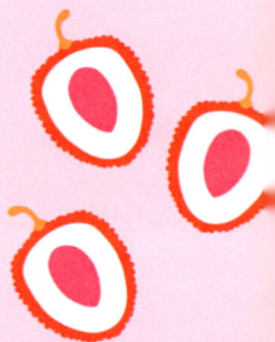

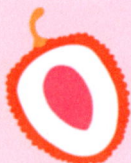

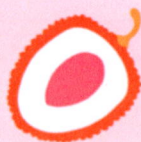

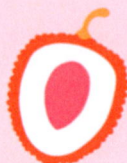

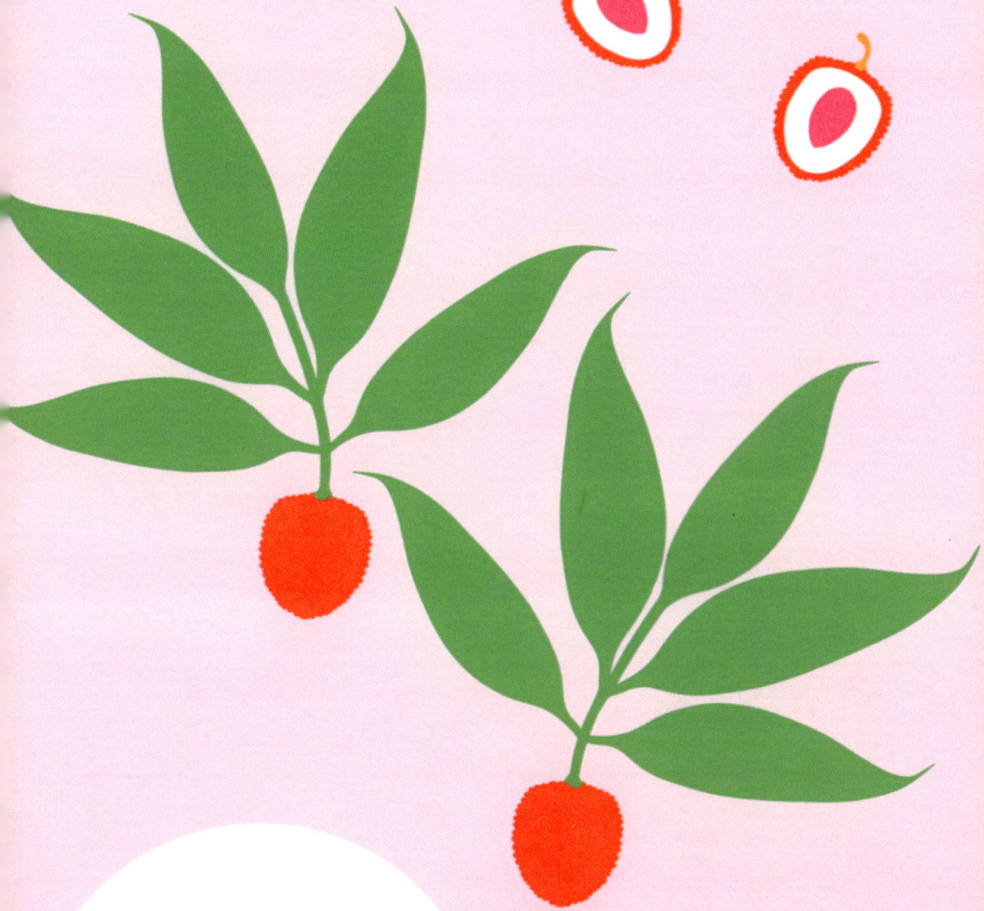

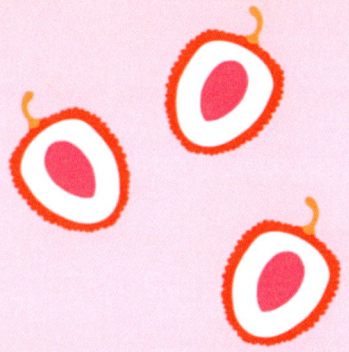

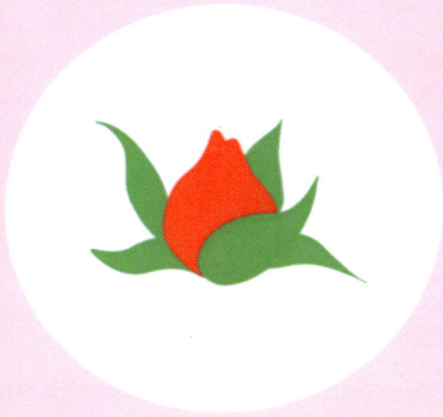

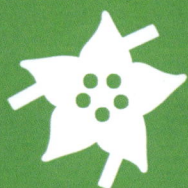

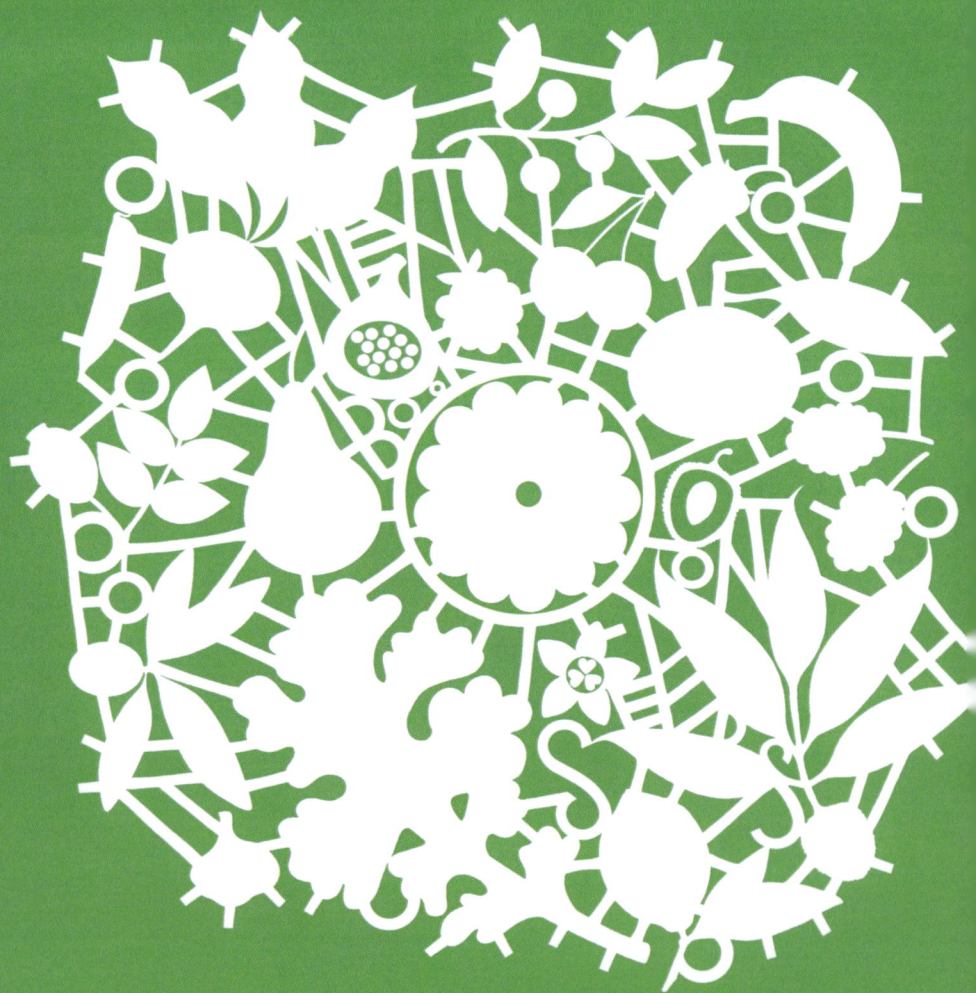

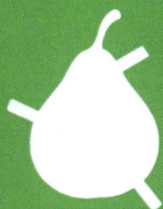

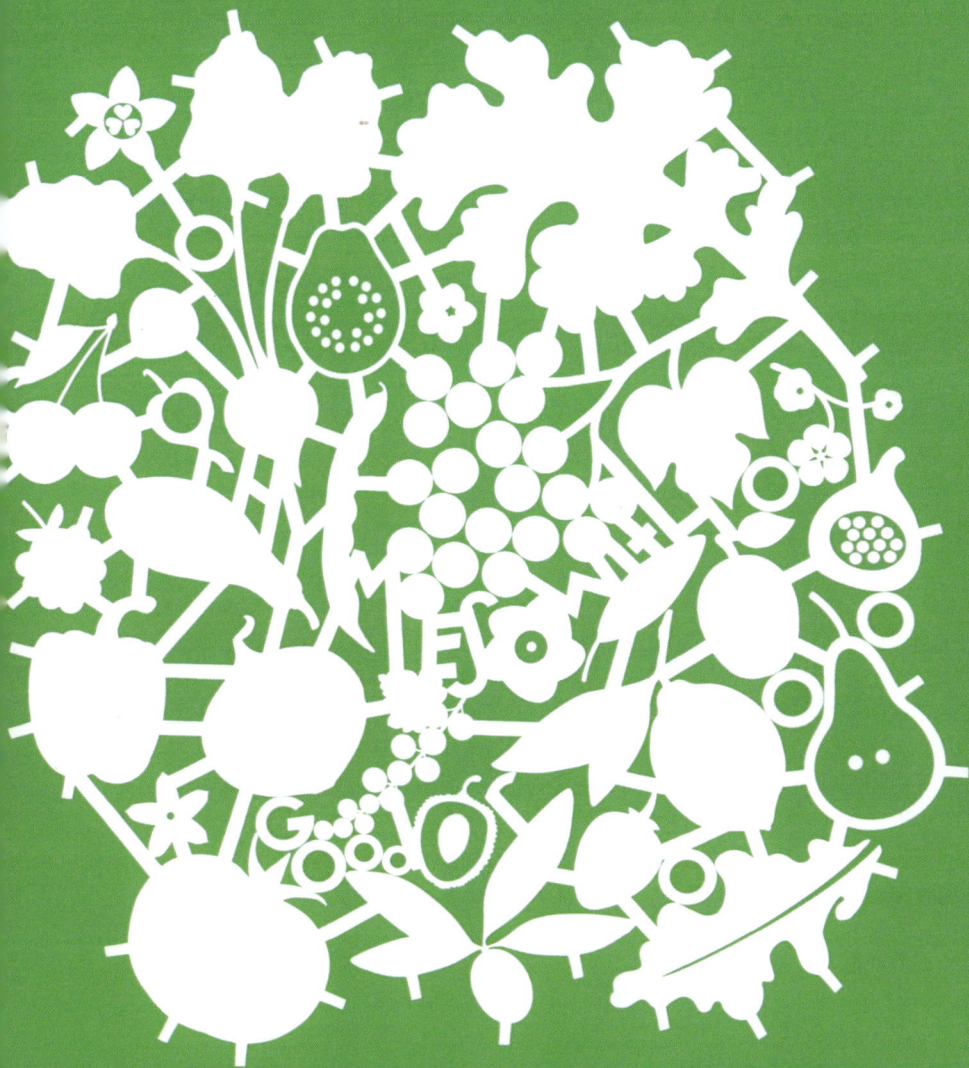

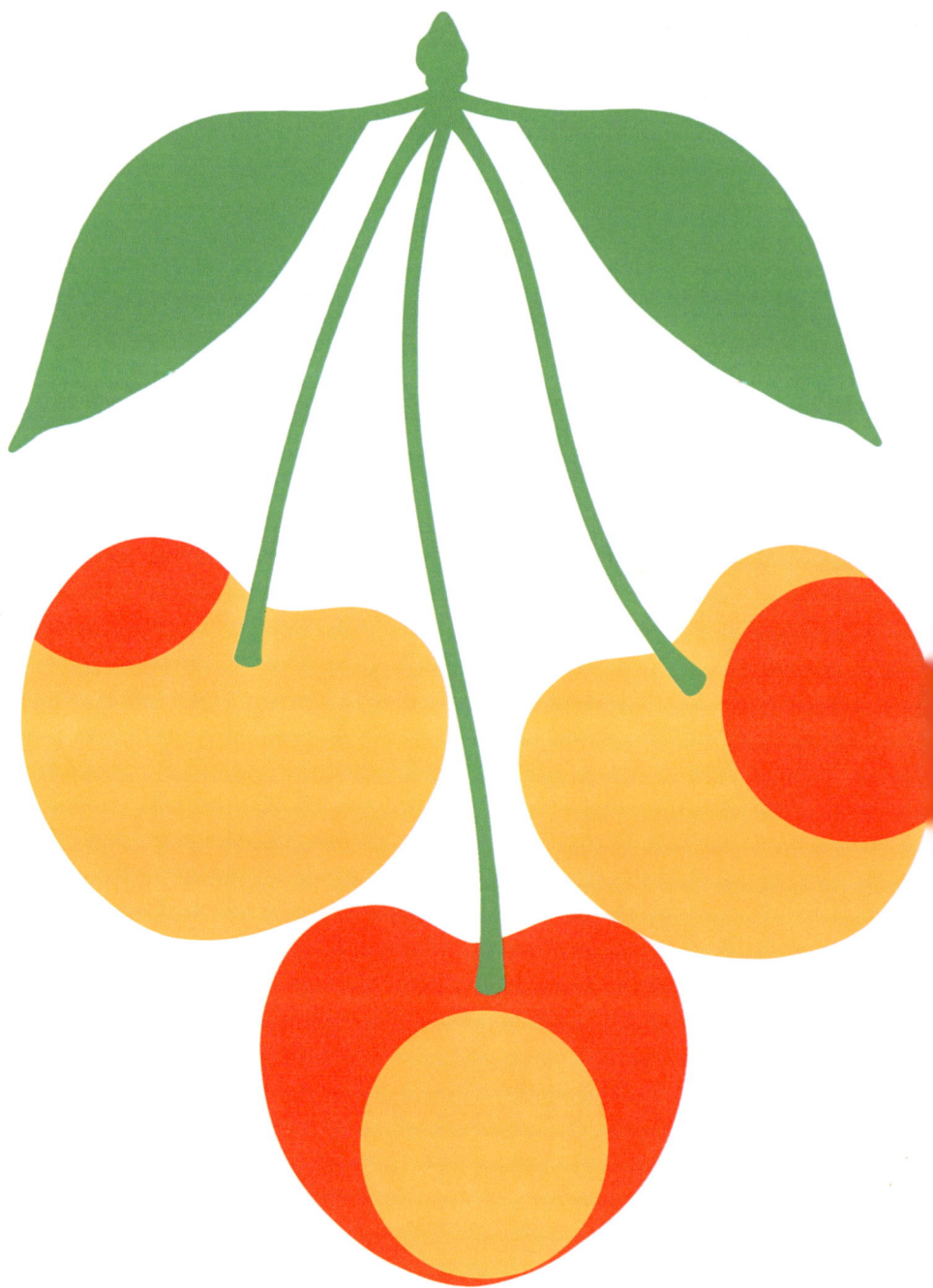

Drink tea at the afterparty.

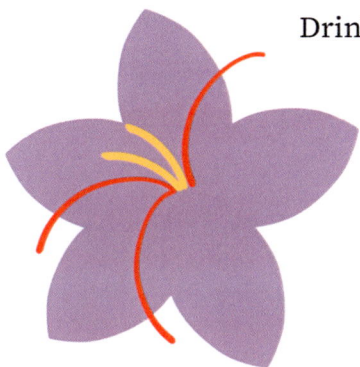

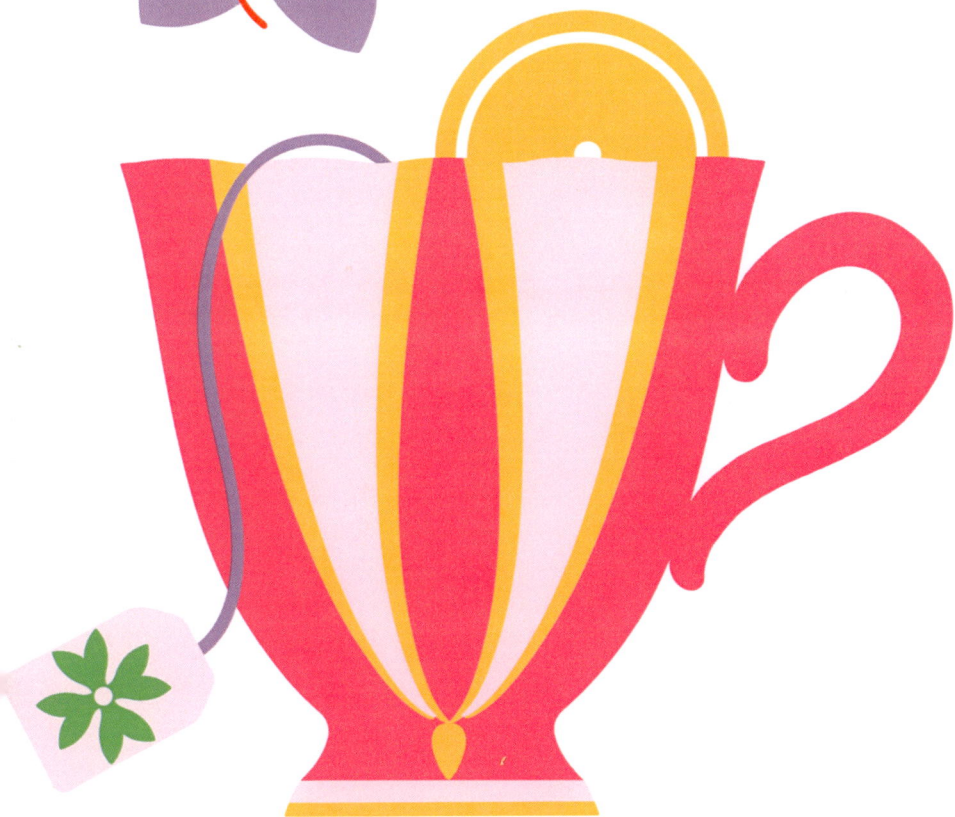

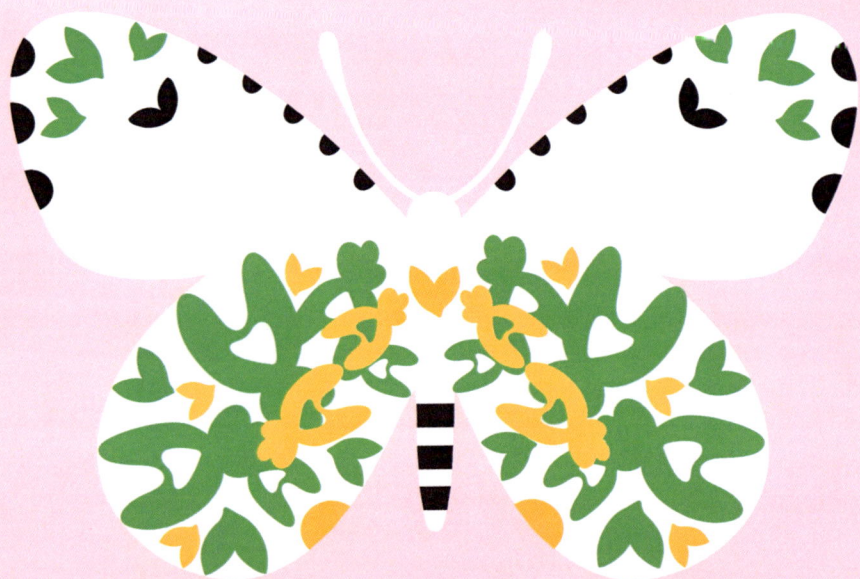